# *10-Minute* CHAIR YOGA EXERCISES FOR SENIORS

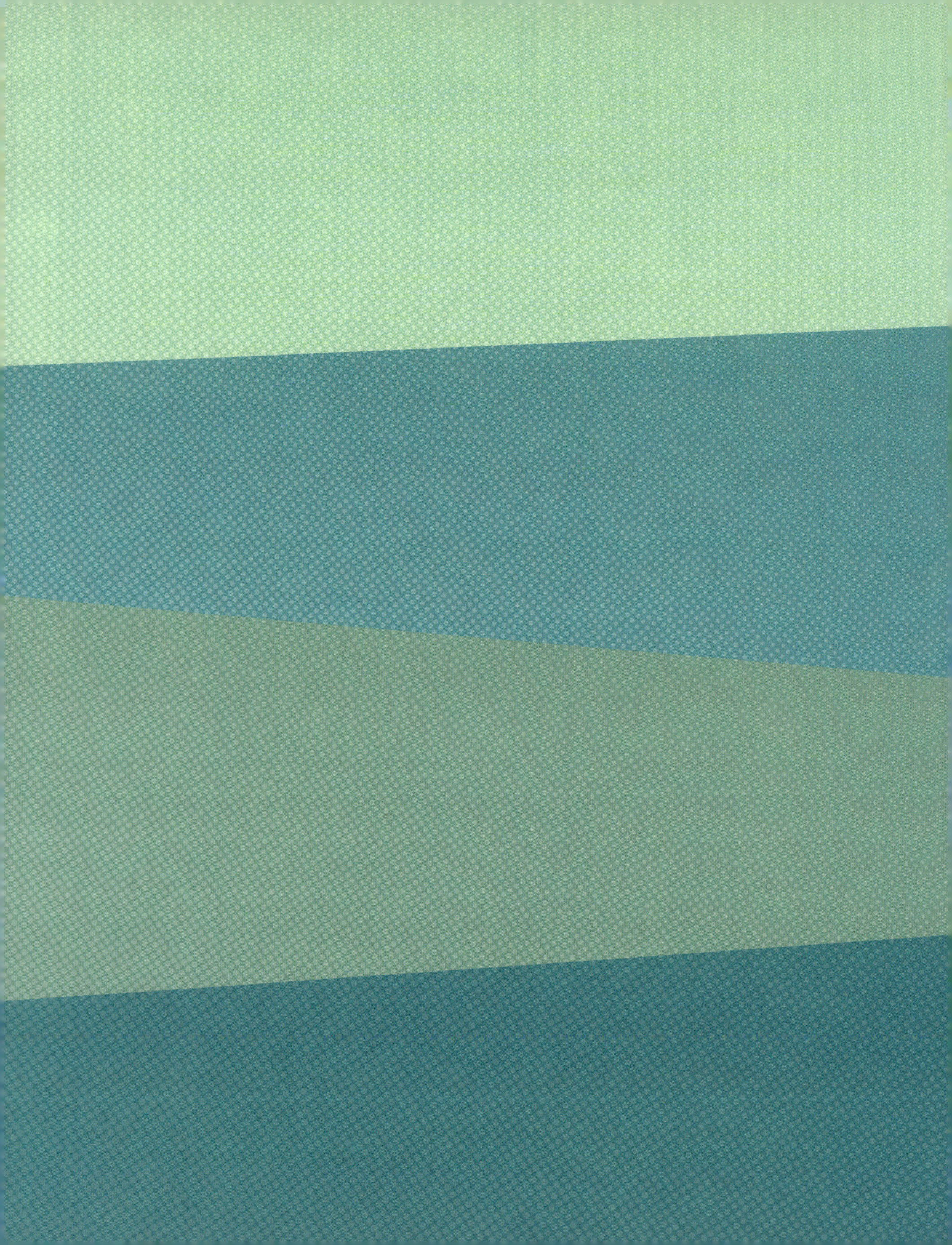

# 10-Minute CHAIR YOGA EXERCISES FOR SENIORS

## 40 Poses to Build Strength and Flexibility for Fall Prevention

APRIL HATTORI

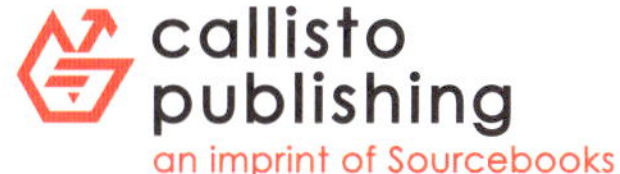

This book is dedicated to my mom, Aiko, who inspires me every day with her beautiful spirit, strength, and sass.

Callisto Publishing LLC

Published by Callisto Publishing LLC C/O Sourcebooks LLC
P.O. Box 4410, Naperville, Illinois 60567-4410
(630) 961-3900
callistopublishing.com


Text by April Hattori
Illustrations by Drew Bardana



Series Designer: Lisa Schreiber
Art Director: Lisa Schreiber
Art Producer: Stacey Stambaugh
Production Editor: Rachel Taenzler
Production Designer: Jeffrey Piekarz



Cataloging-in-Publication Data is on file with the Library of Congress.

Printed and bound in China.
OGP 10 9 8 7 6 5 4 3 2 1

# Contents

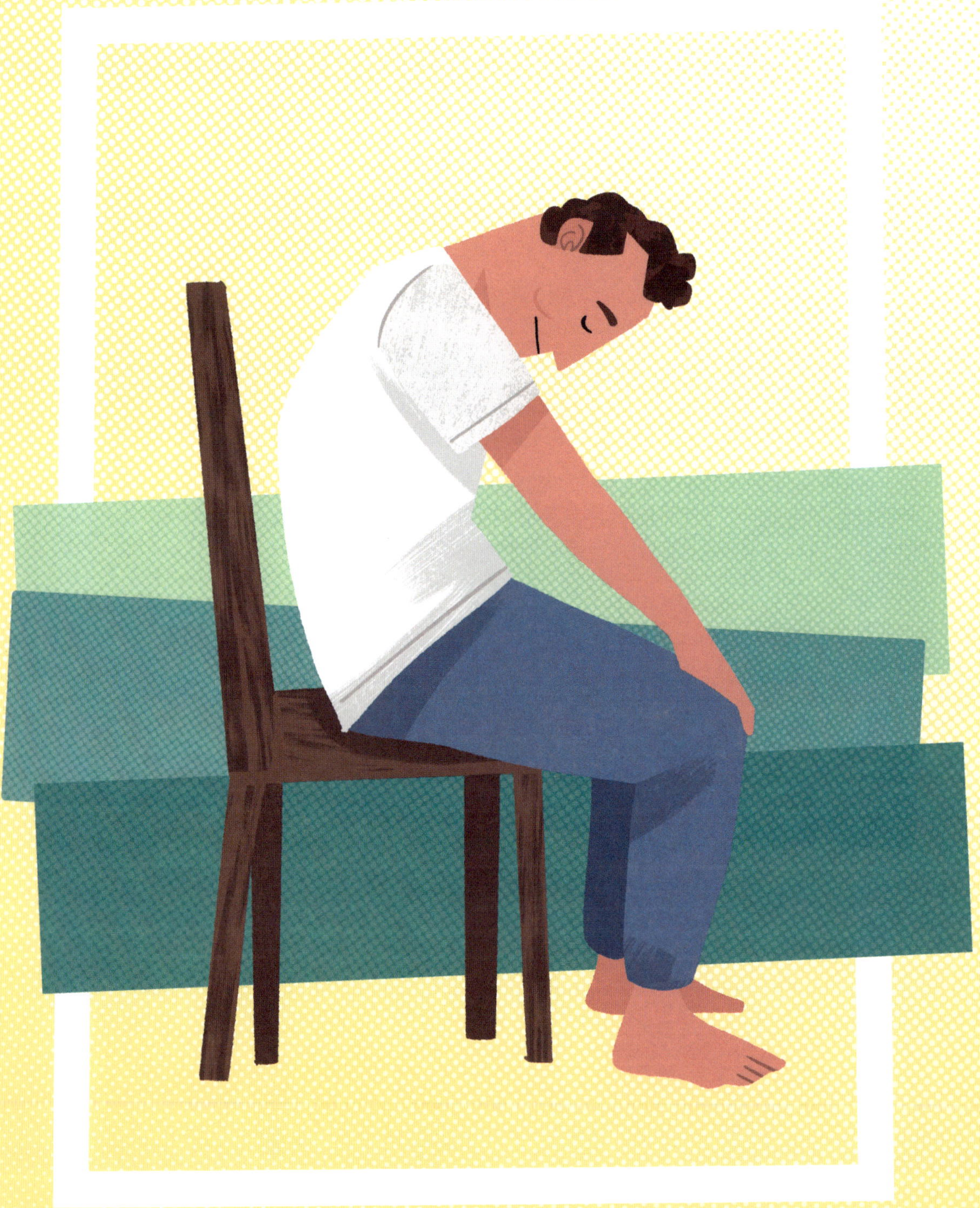

PART ONE

# BUILDING STRENGTH AND FLEXIBILITY

**CONGRATULATIONS** on making a commitment to get healthier by picking up this book! If your goal is to stay strong to enjoy the activities you love, making chair yoga part of your daily routine can be a game changer.

Yoga has been part of my life for more than forty years. As a teenager, after hearing that yoga can enhance flexibility and strength, I enrolled in a class to improve my running. It did that and more. After my first class, feeling refreshed in both body and mind, I was hooked. This passion led me to become a fitness trainer and yoga instructor.

My own journey with yoga over the years inspired me to help older adults, including my eighty-four-year-old mom, get stronger and healthier. I learned that modifying yoga poses so they can be done with a chair made the ancient practice accessible to all—anyone, despite their previous experience with exercise, could improve their strength, flexibility, and balance in a gentle way. My mom has given her stamp of approval to all the poses in this book, using many of the provided modifications to suit her range of motion and ability. I'm thrilled to welcome you into the world of chair yoga—a practice that can help you feel strong in mind, body, and spirit.

## WHAT IS CHAIR YOGA?

Chair yoga is literally yoga—a program of movements and poses, connected to intentional breathing, that gently stretches and strengthens different muscle groups—done with a chair. For older adults, chair yoga is a great way to increase mobility and muscle endurance, improve balance and posture, reduce aches and pains, and boost mood.

Some people may not view yoga as a viable exercise program for a number of reasons. They might think they're too old to start yoga, that chair-supported poses are not effective, or that chair yoga is too easy, but these commonly held beliefs are merely myths.

First, the gentle exercises covered in this book are specifically designed to help individuals of all ages and fitness levels build strength and flexibility gradually and safely. It's never too late to begin movements that stretch and strengthen your muscles while promoting calm and peace.

Second, these exercises are variations of traditional poses—with the support of a chair, you will engage the same muscles and practice the same deep, intentional breathing as in conventional yoga. Chair yoga offers a way to work out every area of your body—there are exercises in this book designed to target your arms, shoulders, core, back, hips, glutes, legs, and feet.

Chair yoga can be as simple or challenging as you want it to be. The routines in this book offer a variety of options to keep your practice engaging, fun, and restorative, including challenge options for each pose.

## THE BENEFITS OF CHAIR YOGA

Doing chair yoga regularly will make you feel stronger and more flexible, which makes your everyday activities easier—everything from hiking to yard work to playing with your grandkids. It also refreshes the mind, bringing serenity and peace to your day. Let's take a closer look at some specific benefits.

## Mobility and Movement

Chair yoga helps counteract the natural decline in muscle mass, flexibility, and bone density that comes with aging. Studies on older adults from support these takeaways: In 2022, Harvard University researchers studying yoga's impact on older adults found improved strength and muscle endurance in participants. And a study at Western University in Canada determined that general exercise and flexibility training can improve flexibility in adults over fifty-five.

## Balance and Fall Prevention

Falls are the leading cause of injuries among older adults. Czech researchers found that yoga improved balance and prevented falls in older adults over age sixty-five, while others at the University of Southern California and the University of California noted a regular yoga practice in older adults led to significant improvements in lower-body strength. Practicing chair yoga strengthens the core and lower-body muscles, and improves flexibility and balance. These benefits are all crucial for stability.

## Relief of Aches and Pains

Like a car racking up miles over the years, our bodies experience natural wear and tear—in the form of joint degeneration, muscle loss, and reduced flexibility—leading to aches, pains, and stiffness. The gentle movements in this book increase circulation and strengthen areas of the body crucial for posture and alignment, allowing your joints to move more effectively.

## Muscle Endurance and Strength

After age thirty, muscle loss can occur at a rate of 3 percent to 5 percent per decade. A 2017 study done at Northumbria University found that physically inactive older adults were more mobile and active after doing chair yoga. Low-impact chair yoga poses that promote an engaged core, such as the Seated Boat pose, gently activate your muscles, helping you stay strong to enjoy the activities you love.

### Joint Health

Exercise is important to keep your joints healthy, even for people with issues such as arthritis. Patients being treated in the hospital for osteoarthritis of the knees and rheumatoid arthritis were found to have benefited from diminished arthritis symptoms through regular yoga practice. A 2018 review of thirteen clinical trials done by several Chinese hospitals—involving 1,557 patients with knee osteoarthritis and rheumatoid arthritis—found that regular yoga practice reduces the symptoms of arthritis. Chair yoga strengthens the muscles around your joints, supporting them better. It can also promote smoother movement by increasing joint lubrication and keeping cartilage healthy through gentle, regular motion.

### Overall Well-being

With its roots tracing back three thousand years, yoga's combination of muscle engagement and relaxation has made this ancient practice a popular way to counter the stress of a busy life. Along with strengthening your body, it's a fantastic way to unwind—whether it's in the morning to start your day, midday to let go of tension, or in the evening to relax before bed. Studies of older adults practicing yoga found not only physical benefits but also improved mental and social well-being.

## GETTING STARTED SAFELY

The poses in this book are designed to challenge your muscles and your willpower. To prevent injury, focus on performing each pose with proper form, and familiarize yourself with the movements before increasing intensity. Using proper form won't just keep you from getting hurt; you'll also get better results as you progress and get stronger and more flexible. Start slowly, listen to your body, and do what feels right for you. This approach will help you build strength safely and steadily.

In our often sedentary lives, many muscles go underused. Chair yoga introduces movements that may feel unfamiliar, as they activate and stretch muscles, tendons, and ligaments that may not have been engaged in a while. It's normal to feel some soreness with new movements—that's your body adapting and getting stronger. If a pose is painful or difficult to sustain, however, don't push through. You can choose to do a more accessible version of the pose or another pose that feels more comfortable. Each pose comes with lower-intensity versions as well as more challenging variations if you've mastered the basics.

## Get Medical Clearance

**The information in this book should not be used in place of the advice of a physician. Before beginning this or any exercise program, please consult with a qualified healthcare provider to get the green light, particularly if you have a condition such as osteoporosis or are recovering from surgery.**

**Experiencing soreness after doing new movements is normal—it means you worked your muscles in a different way. Soreness can come in the form of a dull ache that should subside in a few days. Allow your body to recover before getting back into it. If you experience sharp pain, however, stop immediately and give yourself time to rest. If the pain persists, consult your healthcare provider.**

# HOW TO USE THIS BOOK

Each of the forty poses in part 2 of this book is presented in an easy-to-understand format with friendly illustrations to keep things fun. Then, in part 3, I'll bring all the poses together in twenty-five 10-minute sequences to make your practice fresh and engaging every day.

## Yoga Poses

This book is designed to enable you to do chair yoga from day 1, with opportunities to challenge yourself when you're ready. The forty individual poses in part 2 can be done in any order, or as part of the twenty-five 10-minute sequences that I've designed for you. Each pose description includes targeted areas (the muscle groups engaged during the pose), reminders and things to keep in mind to help your form, modifications to make the pose easier or more challenging, and illustrations showing how to do each step.

## Sequences

The twenty-five sequences in part 3 are designed with goals in mind: There are sequences for mobility, joint health, balance, and more. To make things easy, illustrations and page numbers of each pose are included with each sequence. To support your practice, I've also included warm-up and cooldown sequences that can be done on their own or paired with any sequence.

Each sequence includes the targeted benefits, a list of the poses, and tips to help you make the most of the sequence.

## Cultivating the Right Environment

Start with the basics: Choose a sturdy, armless chair like a dining or folding chair, and wear comfortable clothing. To prevent the chair from sliding, position it against a wall and/or on a nonslip surface such as a yoga mat or rug with a mat. If your feet don't reach the floor, place a pillow or folded towel or blanket under them to create a stable base. While yoga is traditionally done barefoot, nonslip socks can be a safe alternative to stabilize your footing.

Creating a peaceful environment for your yoga practice will help you fully benefit from each pose. If possible, create a dedicated, distraction-free space in your home. To deepen your relaxation, consider adding soft lighting and/or peaceful music to create a soothing atmosphere and ease you into your practice.

## CREATING A REGULAR YOGA PRACTICE

In his book *Light on Life*, yogi B. K. S. Iyengar wrote, "The moment you bring attention, you are creating something, and creation has life and energy." By choosing to make yoga part of your day, you are improving your life on many levels, including increased strength and a calm mind. Yoga can energize your morning, relieve midday stress, and help you unwind before bed.

To stay motivated, try tracking your sessions—whether on a paper calendar or using an app. Reflect on how you feel after each practice. Celebrate the small victories, such as reduced soreness or improved flexibility, and treat yourself with positive rewards. After an evening practice, I like to enjoy a cup of peppermint or chamomile tea.

The beauty of chair yoga is that perfection is not the priority. The goals are to be present in your practice and to do your best.

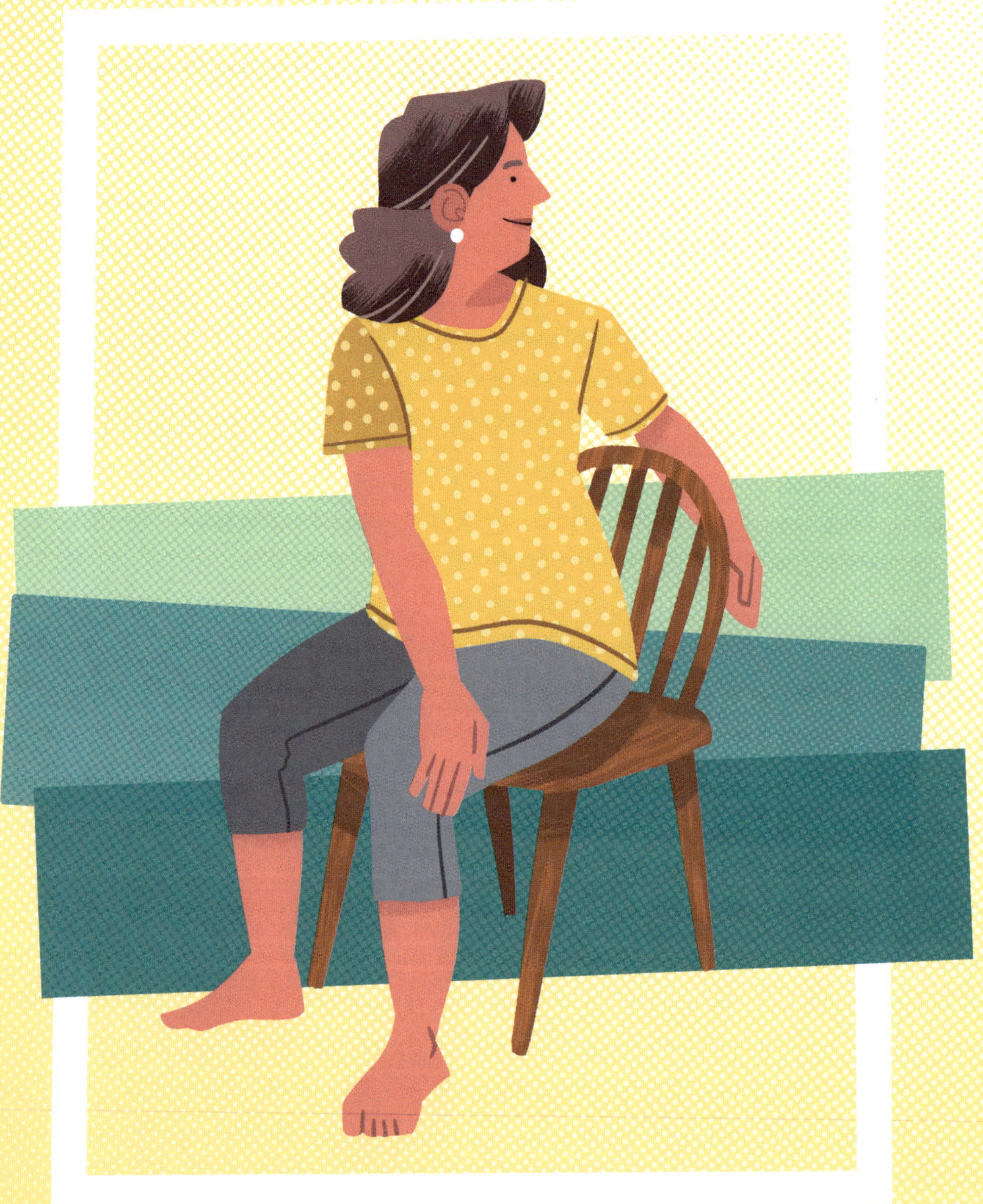

PART TWO

# CHAIR YOGA POSES

**LET'S HAVE SOME FUN** and strike a pose with chair yoga! Each pose in this section comes with cheerful illustrations, easy-to-follow steps, tips, modifications, and a rundown of the muscles you're giving a little love. The poses are grouped by the muscles they work—upper body, lower body, core, and the whole body—so you can target what you need most. You can do the poses on their own, mix and match, or follow the ready-made sequences in part 3 once you have a handle on the movements (page 91).

Don't forget to breathe! Deep breathing is a key part of yoga. Try this: Inhale deeply through your nose, like you're filling your belly with air, and exhale slowly through your nose or mouth. This method gets your diaphragm—the star of your breathing muscles—working its magic to fill your lungs properly.

Ready to get started? Begin your practice with a gentle warm-up (page 92) to wake up your body and set the stage for a great session. Let's get moving!

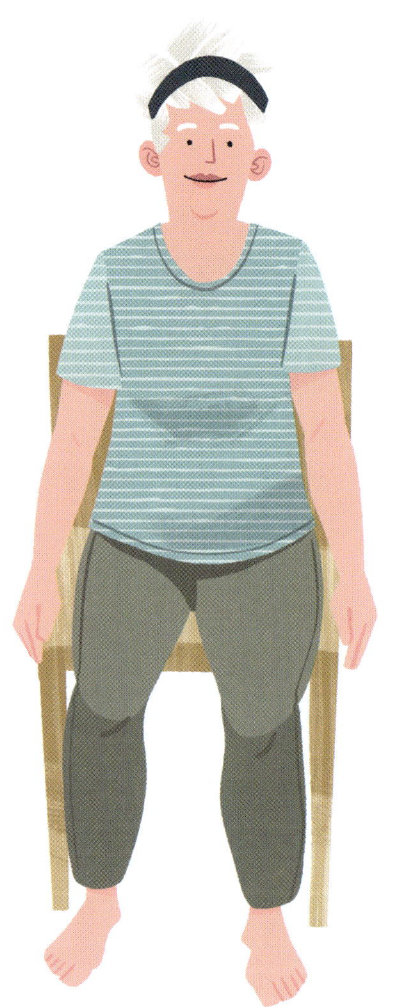

**REMEMBER**

Sit tall, pulling your belly button in toward your spine and activating your core. Imagine a string at the top of your head pulling you upward. Gaze forward with your neck straight, centered over the middle of your chest.

# SEATED MOUNTAIN

## TADASANA

**TARGETED AREAS:** Arms, back, core, feet, hips, shoulders

Seated Mountain will enhance your posture and core stability while gently improving flexibility in your shoulders and arms. This pose is the starting point and transition for many poses, and it will help you connect your breathing to your movement in a way that provides a foundation for the other poses. With practice, this pose can also enhance proprioception, or bodily awareness.

### INSTRUCTIONS

1. Sit tall toward the front edge of your chair with your feet flat on the floor, hip-width apart, knees over ankles. Press strongly into both feet—big toe, little toe, and the center of the heel. Keep your shoulders soft and open your chest slightly—imagine broadening the space between your collarbones.
2. Let your arms hang at your sides with your palms facing inward with fingers spread, reaching toward the floor.
3. Take 3 to 5 rounds of breath.

To simplify, rest your hands on your thighs.

For a challenge, stand up. With your feet hip-width apart, grip the back of the chair with one hand for stability.

In both the seated and standing variations, you can engage your leg muscles more by placing your feet and knees together.

**Keep in Mind:** You should feel equal weight distributed in your feet. Focus on sitting or standing tall and keeping your head back with your ears over your shoulders, gently bringing your shoulders back and down. This will naturally help you avoid slouching and rounding your shoulders.

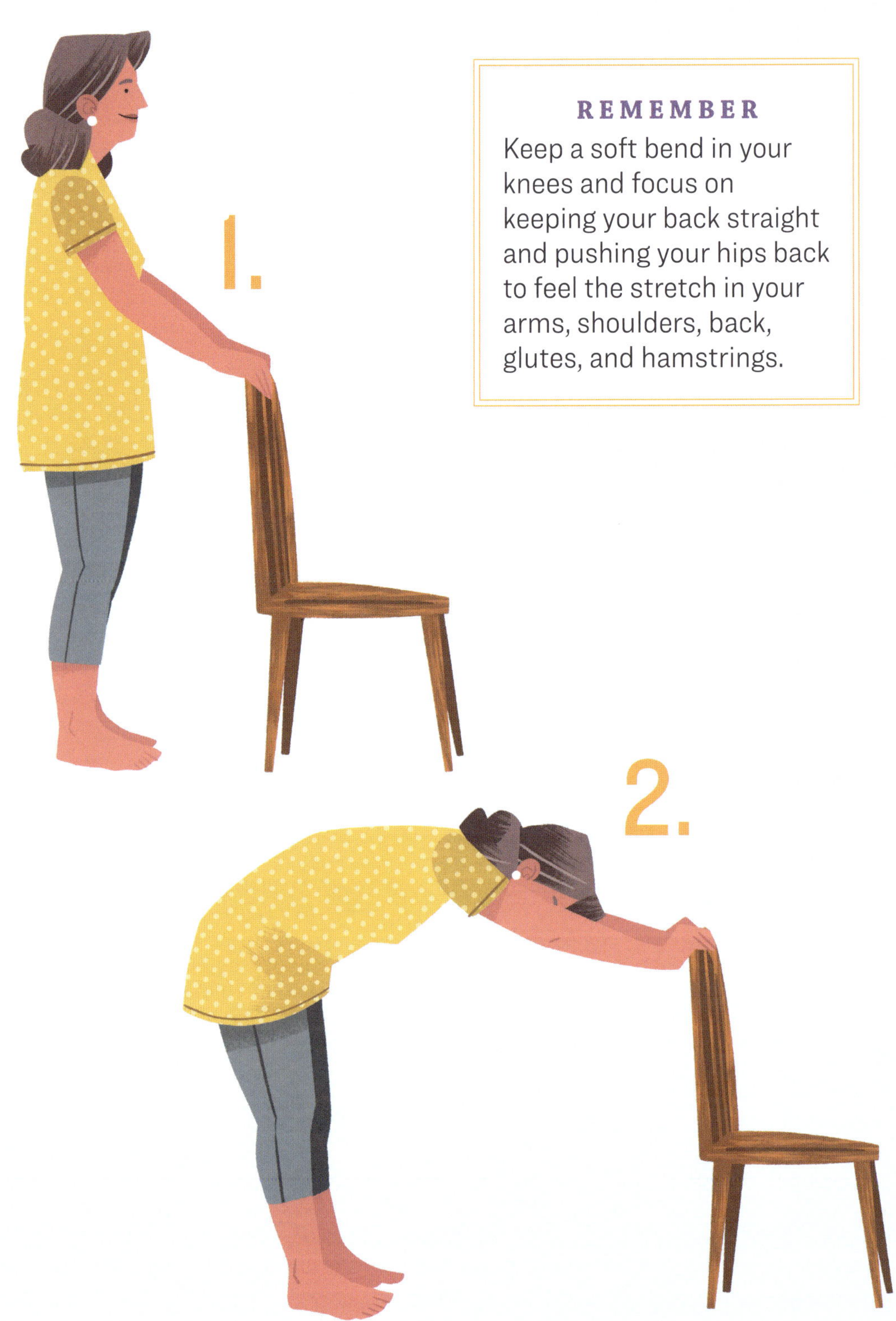


**REMEMBER**

Keep a soft bend in your knees and focus on keeping your back straight and pushing your hips back to feel the stretch in your arms, shoulders, back, glutes, and hamstrings.

# STANDING DOWNWARD DOG

## ADHO MUKHA SVANASANA

**TARGETED AREAS:** Back, calves, hamstrings, shoulders

Downward Dog is one of my favorite poses, especially when I'm short on time and want to release tension in my neck and back. It's a full-body stretch that improves flexibility, mobility, and strength, enhancing balance and helping you reach overhead with ease.

### INSTRUCTIONS

1. Stand 2 to 3 feet from the back of the chair, feet hip-width apart. Inhale and place your hands on the back of the chair.
2. Exhale, step back, and bend at the hips with your arms straight and a soft bend in your elbows and knees.
3. Take 3 to 5 rounds of breath and come up to a standing position slowly.

To simplify, skip the chair and use a wall. Find a comfortable height for your hands to rest and explore a gentle stretch with more support.

For a challenge, place your hands on the seat of the chair to deepen the stretch.

**Keep in Mind:** If you have neck or spine issues, high blood pressure, eye pressure conditions, balance challenges, or other health issues, consult with your healthcare professional before doing this pose. It may be best to keep your neck aligned with your spine and your head higher or level with your heart.

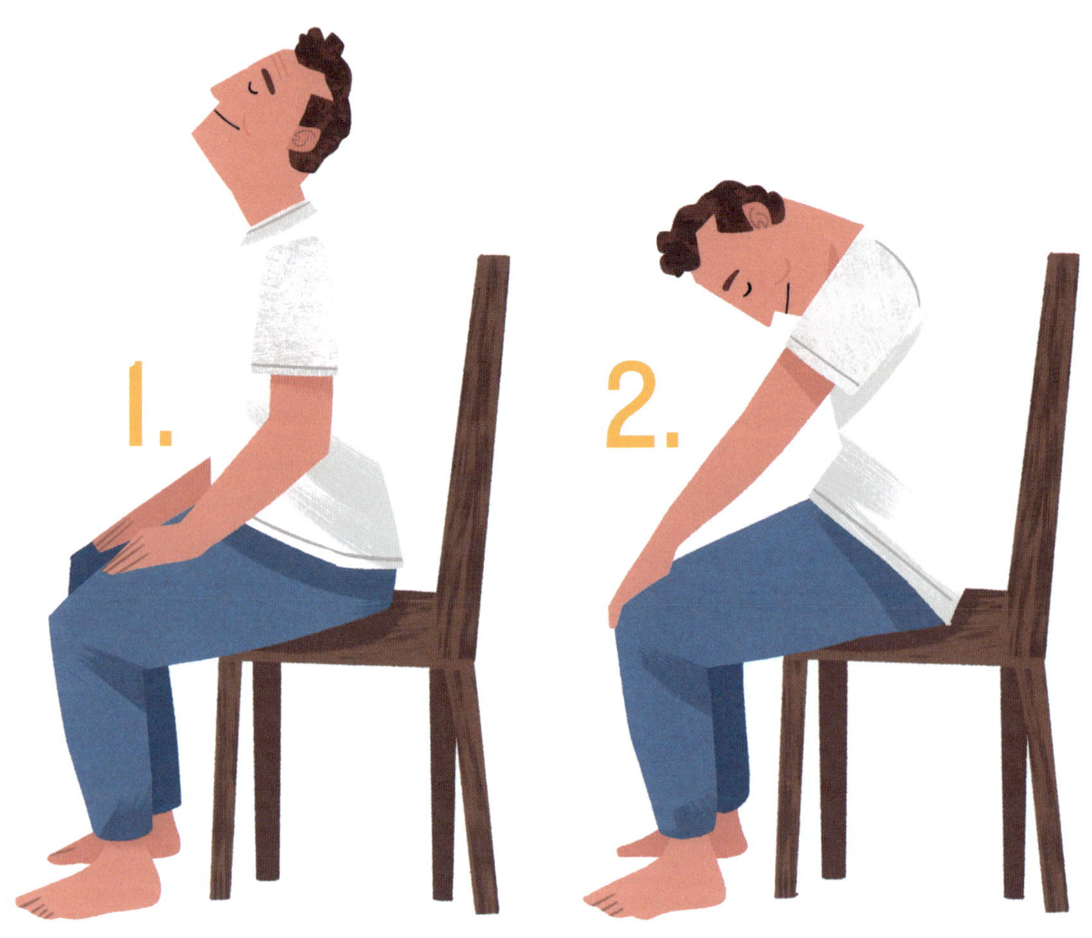


**REMEMBER**

In "Cat," let your tailbone start the motion of the arch rather than forcing your neck or back. Let that motion gradually travel your spine up to your neck. Don't lead by tipping your head back to start the pose.

# SEATED CAT-COW

## MARJAYASANA (CAT), BITILASANA (COW)

**TARGETED AREAS:** Back/spine, core, neck

A flexible back is important for every movement that we do, even something like bending down to tie our shoes. Seated Cat-Cow gently mobilizes the spine with an easy breathing pattern—you inhale in "Cow" and exhale in "Cat," synchronized with the arching and rounding of your spine.

### INSTRUCTIONS

1. From Seated Mountain (page 10), inhale and start "Cow" by arching your back, tilting the top of your pelvis forward, and bringing your shoulder blades together while lifting your chest and gazing slightly upward. Imagine creating a gentle convex curve from your tailbone to your neck.
2. Exhale into "Cat," dropping your chin toward your chest and rounding your back. Gently tilt your hips under so your tailbone points slightly downward while drawing your belly button to your spine.
3. Repeat this sequence 3 to 5 times.

To simplify, sit tall with your back straight and focus on breathing: Inhale deeply to expand the chest (as in "Cow") and exhale to relax the back (as in "Cat").

For a challenge, as you start "Cow," sweep your arms out to the side and up, bringing your palms together overhead. As you start "Cat," bring your hands out in front of you to hold. Lifting your feet off the floor even for a second can engage your core more.

**Keep in Mind:** If you have spinal issues and/or osteoporosis, consult with your healthcare professional before doing this pose. If you have back or neck issues, round and arch your spine only as much as is comfortable for you, focusing on smaller, controlled movement.

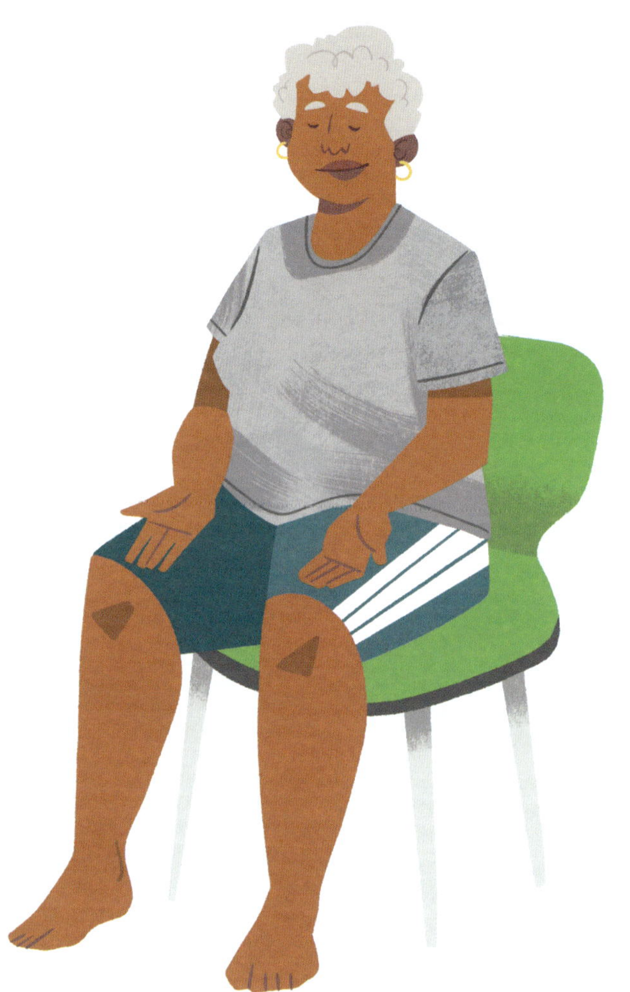

**REMEMBER**

Bring awareness to your entire body, scanning from head to toe, releasing tension in each area as you exhale.

# SEATED REST

## SAVASANA

**TARGETED AREAS:** Core, total body awareness

Seated Rest is the perfect way to soothe your mind and body after an energizing yoga session. To maximize relaxation, focus on breathing deeply, feeling your belly expand as your diaphragm contracts, allowing air into your lungs.

### INSTRUCTIONS

1. Let your back rest against the back of the chair, allowing your body to relax.
2. Let your legs and feet rest naturally. Rest your hands on your thighs, palms facing up. Close your eyes and soften your face, including your jaw and around your eyes.
3. Inhale slowly and deeply through your nose and exhale gently through your nose or mouth. Stay in this position for 1 to 3 minutes.

For a challenge, sit at the edge of the front of your chair without reclining and focus on engaging your core to maintain an upright posture. Lift your arms slightly away from your thighs, palms facing up.

**Keep in Mind:** Make sure your feet are supported to avoid strain on your lower back and hips.

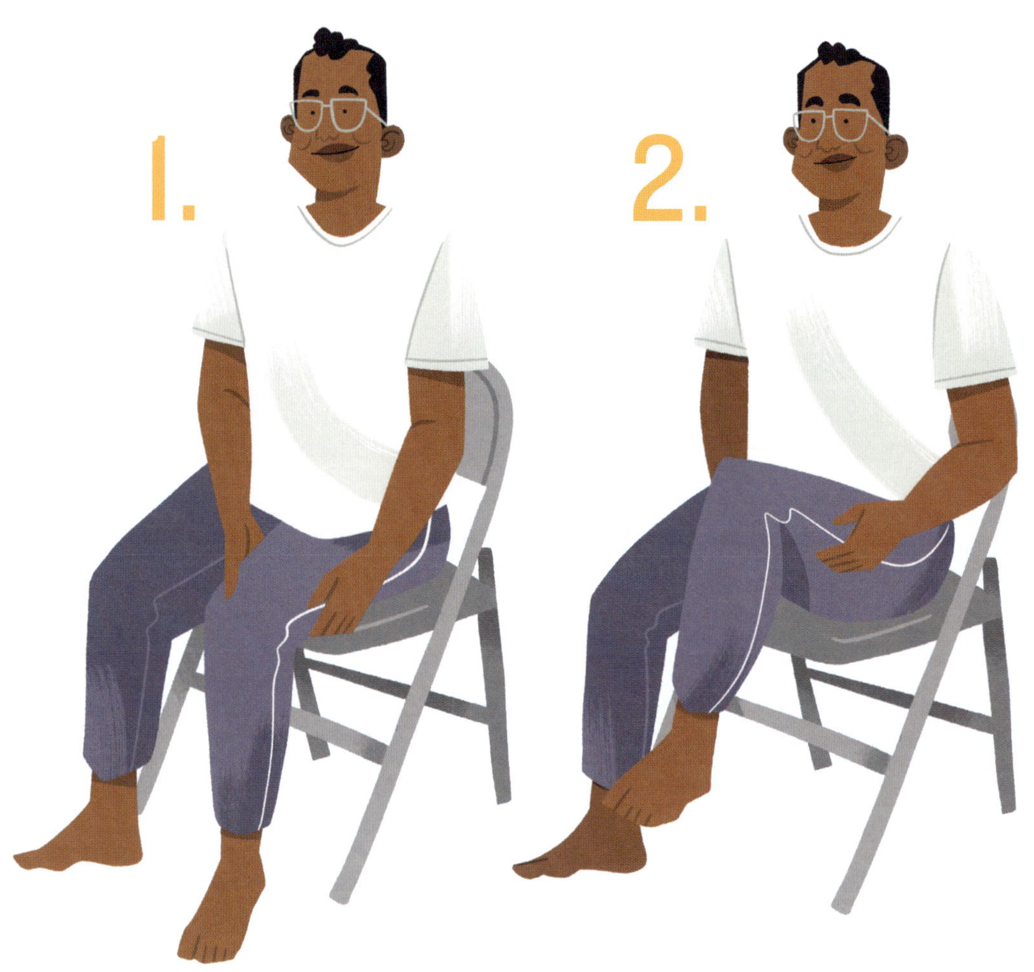


**REMEMBER**

Sit tall and keep your core engaged by pulling your belly button toward your spine.

# SEATED LOW LUNGE

## ANJANEYASANA

**TARGETED AREAS:** Core, glutes, hip flexors, knees

When it comes to walking with ease and staying mobile, lower-body flexibility is just as important as building muscle. Seated Low Lunge stretches the glutes and strengthens your hip muscles while improving posture and strengthening your core.

### INSTRUCTIONS

1. From Seated Mountain (page 10), inhale and place the fingers of both hands under each side of your right thigh.
2. Using your hands, exhale and gently lift your right knee toward your chest. Hold this position for 3 to 5 rounds of breath while maintaining an upright posture.
3. Lower your leg back to the starting position. Focus on stretching your spine upward to maintain a tall and aligned posture.
4. Repeat with the left leg.

To simplify, use a belt or dish towel for support by placing it under your thigh, holding each side with one hand, and lifting.

For a challenge, lift your leg without using your hands for support. Flex your ankle to engage your legs more.

**Keep in Mind:** If you feel tightness in your back thigh or glute, do not attempt to lift your knee any higher, bringing it to a comfortable place instead. To protect your spine and strengthen your core, do not round your back or lean back as you lift your knee to a comfortable level.

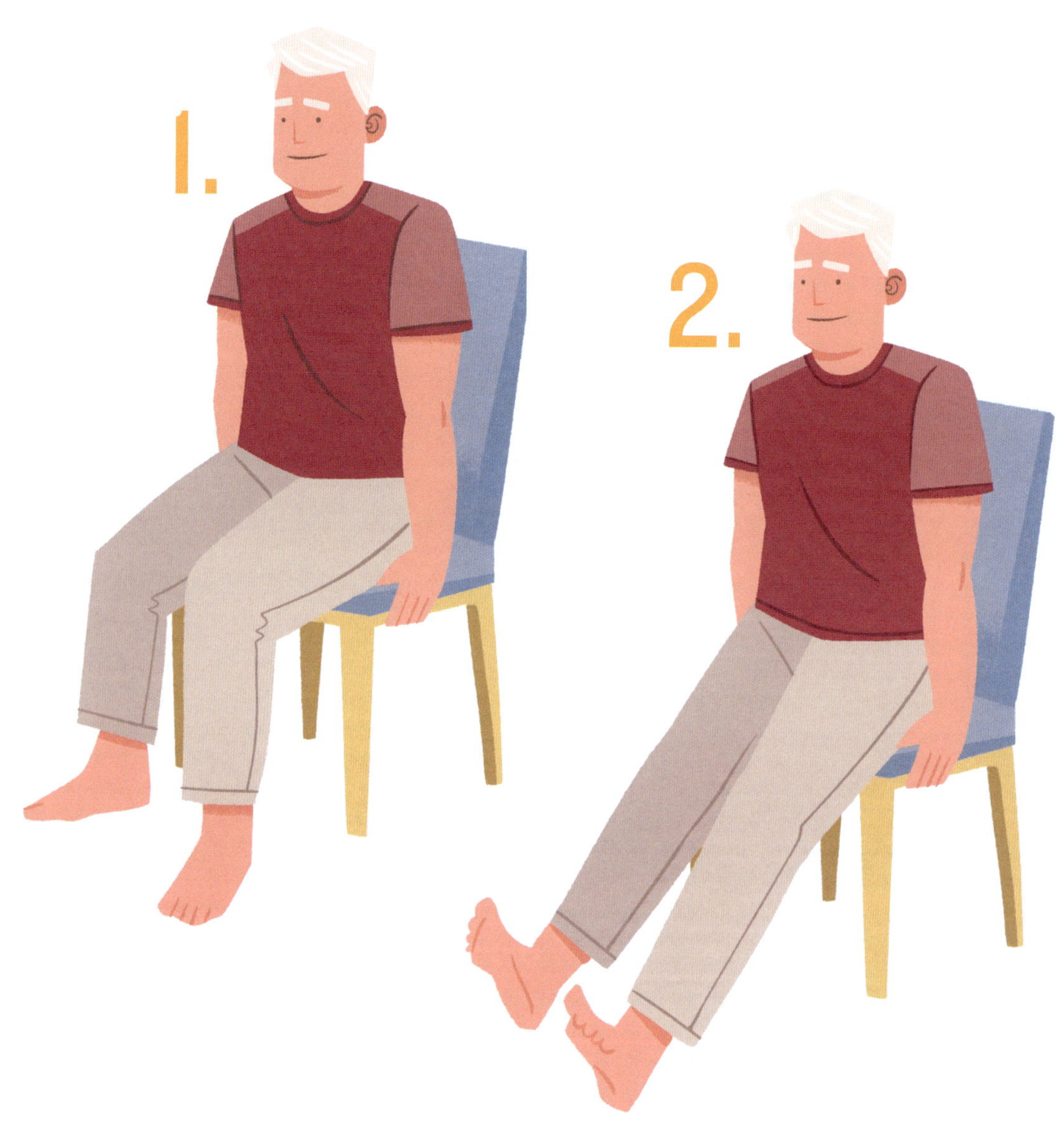


**REMEMBER**

Keep a soft bend in your knees and activate your front thighs.

# SEATED STAFF

## DANDASANA

**TARGETED AREAS:** Core, hamstrings, hip flexors, quadriceps

Seated Staff is incredibly versatile—it's easy to do at home, in a car, even an airplane if you don't have anything under the seat in front of you! This pose strengthens your legs, stretches your calves and ankles, and engages your core. It's great for building balance.

## INSTRUCTIONS

1. Sit toward the front of your chair and place your hands at the sides of the chair.
2. Inhale and straighten your legs, engaging your thighs, while pressing your heels into the floor and flexing your ankles, drawing your toes back toward your face and feeling your kneecaps lift.
3. Exhale, pressing your hands firmly on the sides of the chair. Hold the position for 3 slow, deep breaths. Maintain steady engagement in your legs, core, and shoulders.

To simplify, keep your feet flat on the floor, knees over ankles. Focus on evenly distributing your weight across the bottom of each foot.

For a challenge, from the main pose, lift your heels slightly off the floor to increase the challenge for your core and legs.

**Keep in Mind:** Keep your back straight and don't round your shoulders, drawing on your core strength to keep your body aligned. If you feel strain in your lower back or hamstrings, bend your knees.

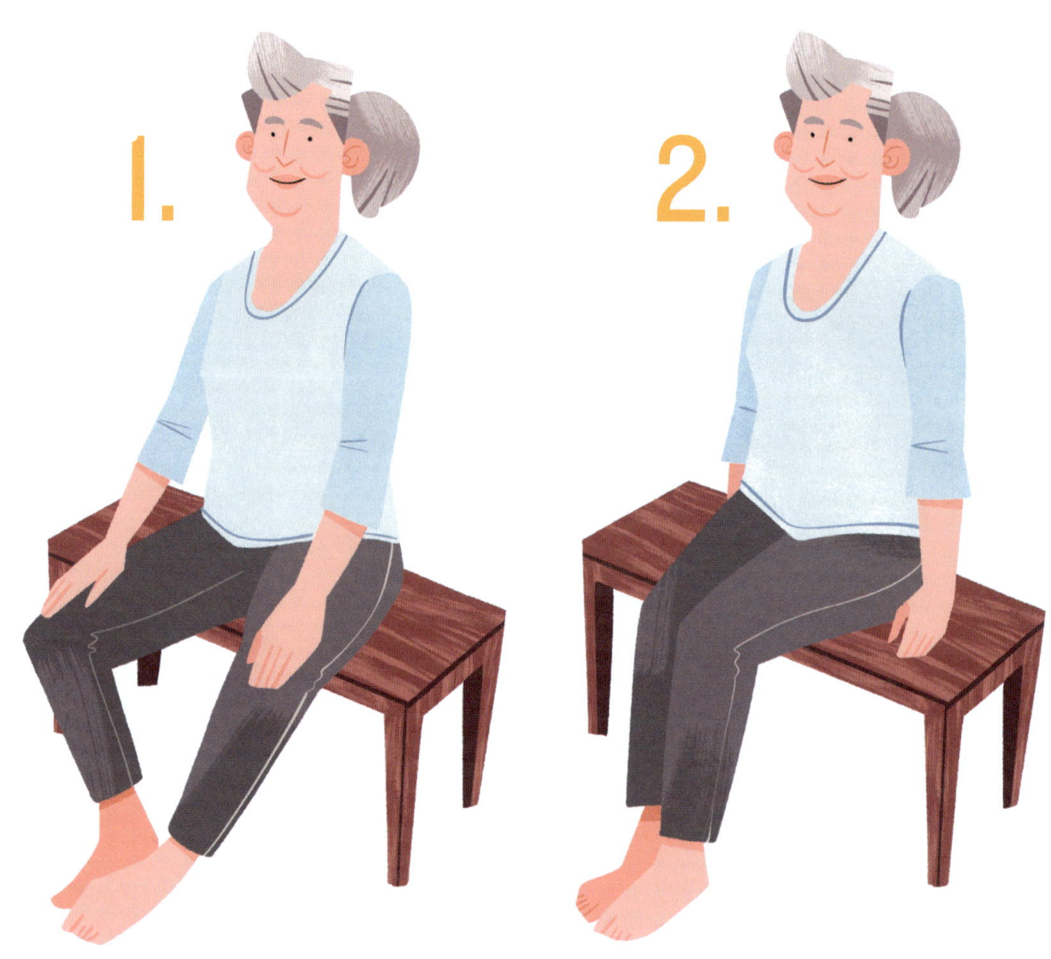


**REMEMBER**

Sit as close to the edge of the chair as you can while keeping your sit bones, or seat, solidly on the chair. This will allow your knees to open more easily.

# SEATED BUTTERFLY

## TITLI ASANA

**TARGETED AREAS:** Groin, hips, thighs

Imagine graceful butterfly wings as you enjoy this active pose. Sitting for long periods, whether at a desk or watching TV, can tighten your hip muscles. This can affect your ability to get on and off the floor or into and out of low chairs. The Seated Butterfly helps gently open your hips, promoting flexibility and ease of movement.

### INSTRUCTIONS

1. Sit tall toward the edge of your chair with the inside of your heels and balls of your feet touching, letting your knees fall open to the sides.
2. Breathe naturally and gently open and close your knees like butterfly wings to loosen the hips. Aim for 10 to 20 repetitions.

To simplify, skip the dynamic flapping motion and simply hold the position with knees open to a comfortable position, focusing on breathing and relaxation.

For a challenge, slide your feet closer to the chair to deepen the stretch, further opening up the hips.

**Keep in Mind:** Skip this pose if you are recovering from procedures such as hip or knee replacements, or if you have acute pain in your hips, knees, or groin, unless cleared by your doctor or physical therapist.

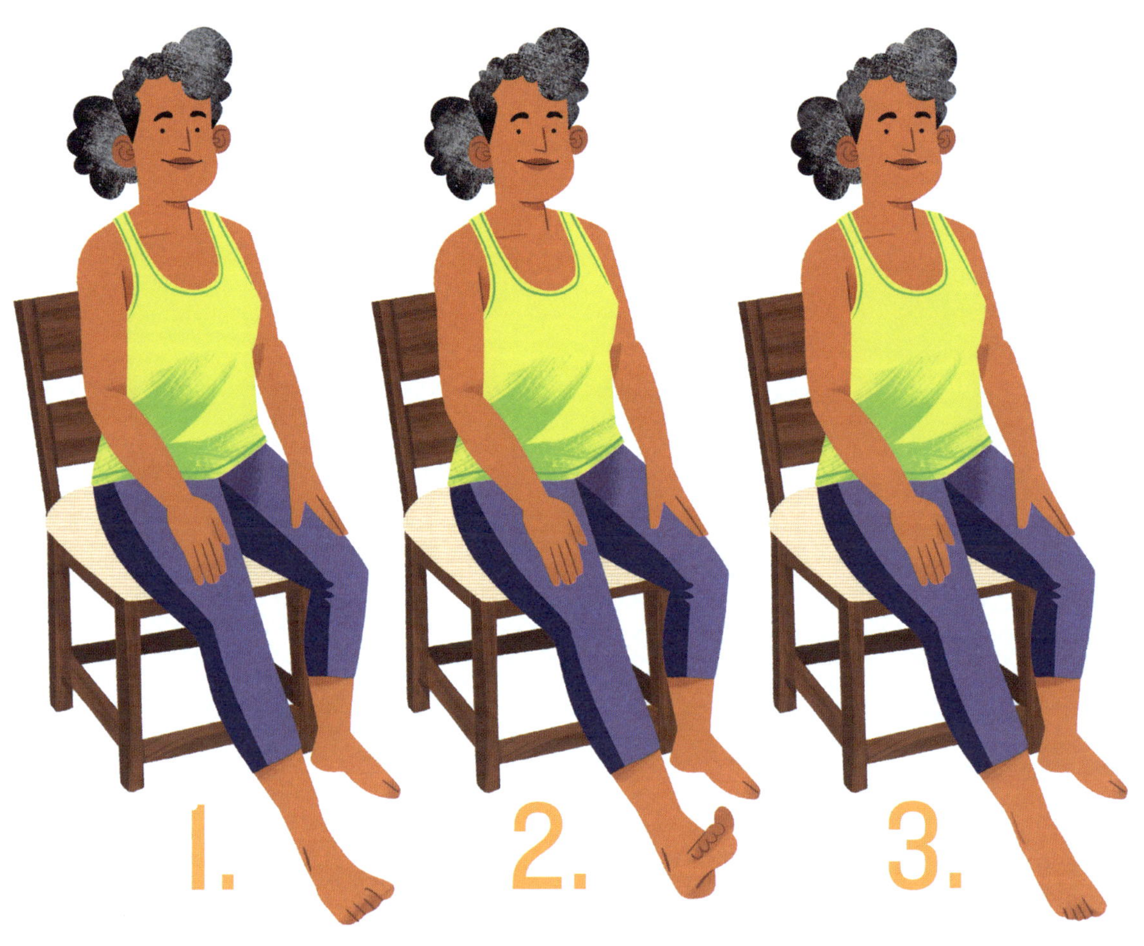


**REMEMBER**

Sit tall to activate your core and support your hips as you activate your lower body.

# SEATED CALF AND TOE STRETCH

## PASCHIMOTTANASANA/ADHO MUKHA SVANASANA

**TARGETED AREAS:** Ankles, calves, feet

Having flexibility in your feet and ankles is important for staying mobile and preventing leg cramps. Flexing and pointing the toes while stretching the legs isolates the toe and calf engagement in poses like Standing Downward Dog (page 12).

### INSTRUCTIONS

1. From Seated Mountain (page 10), fully extend one leg forward, resting your heel on the floor.
2. Inhale and extend your ankle, pointing your toes away from you. Hold for 2 seconds.
3. Exhale and flex your ankle, toes pulled toward your head. Keep breathing through the hold.
4. Repeat sequence 5 to 10 times and switch to other leg.

To simplify, keep your foot flat on the floor, knee over ankle. Flex and extend your ankle, toes up and down.

For a challenge, make small circles with your big toe, mobilizing your ankle. After five to ten circles, repeat in the other direction, then switch feet.

**Keep in Mind:** Focus on moving within a comfortable range of motion. To avoid straining your joints, tendons, or muscles, do not overextend your ankle by flexing or pointing your foot too far or lock your knee.

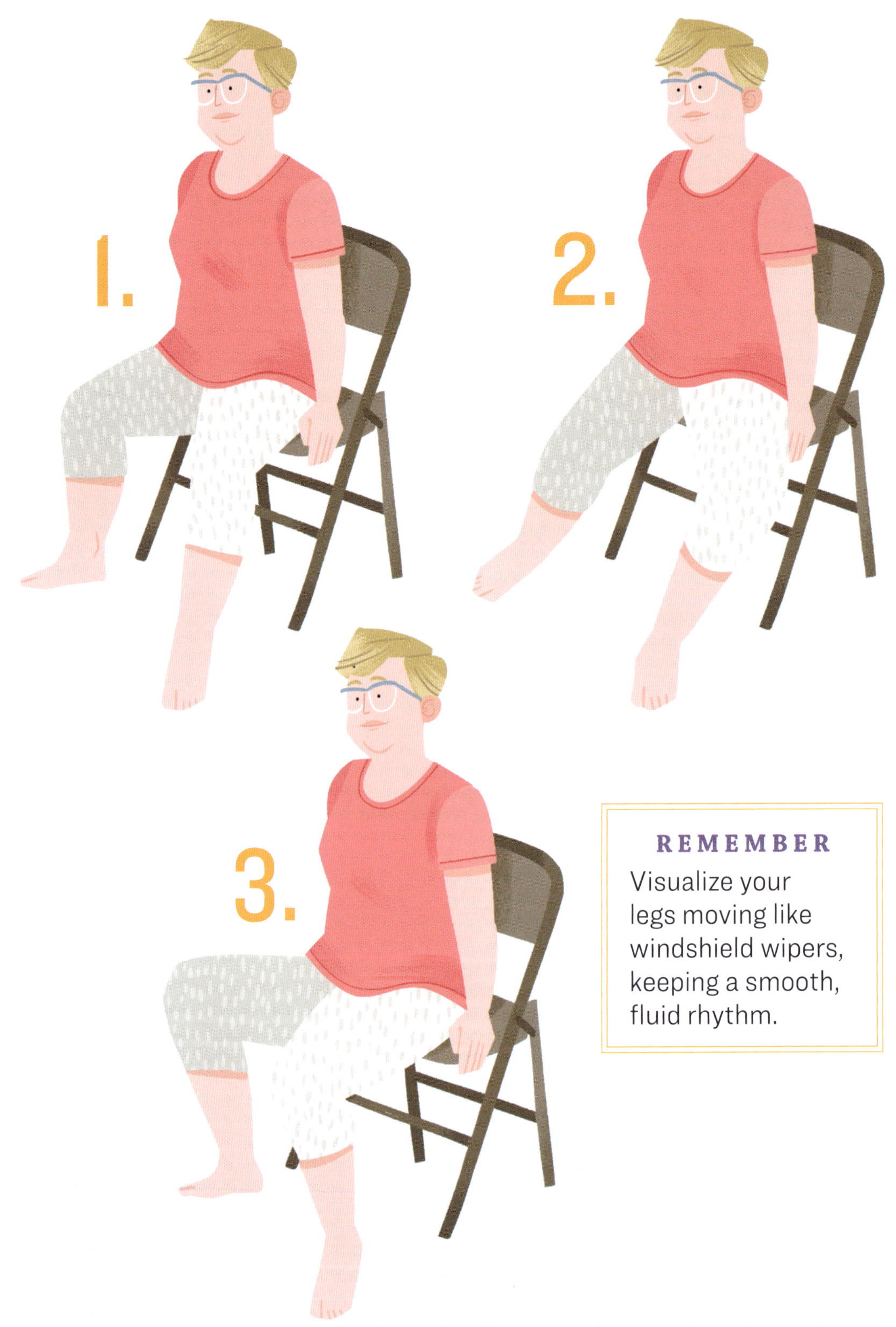


**REMEMBER**

Visualize your legs moving like windshield wipers, keeping a smooth, fluid rhythm.

# SEATED WINDSHIELD WIPER

## SUPTA MATSYENDRASANA

**TARGETED AREAS:** Core, glutes, hips, thighs

Clean out those hip cobwebs with the Seated Windshield Wiper, a dynamic pose that eases lower back tension, helps with arthritis, and can improve circulation and hip joint health. It can help you stay mobile and strong with everyday movements like walking or turning.

### INSTRUCTIONS

1. Inhale and sit up straight with your hips closer to the edge of your chair with feet flat on the floor and wider than hip-width apart. Place your hands on the sides of the chair or on your thighs.
2. Exhale while dropping your knees to the right, inhale while moving them back center.
3. Exhale, dropping your knees to the left. Your feet will pivot slightly as you move.
4. Do 5 to 10 times each direction.

To simplify, hold your knees to one side for three to five rounds of breath and switch to the other side.

For a challenge, as you let your knees drop to one side, twist your torso in the opposite direction, reaching the opposite arm across your body.

**Keep in Mind:** Move within your range of motion, being careful not to over-stretch. If you have hip issues or surgeries, check with your healthcare professional before doing this movement.

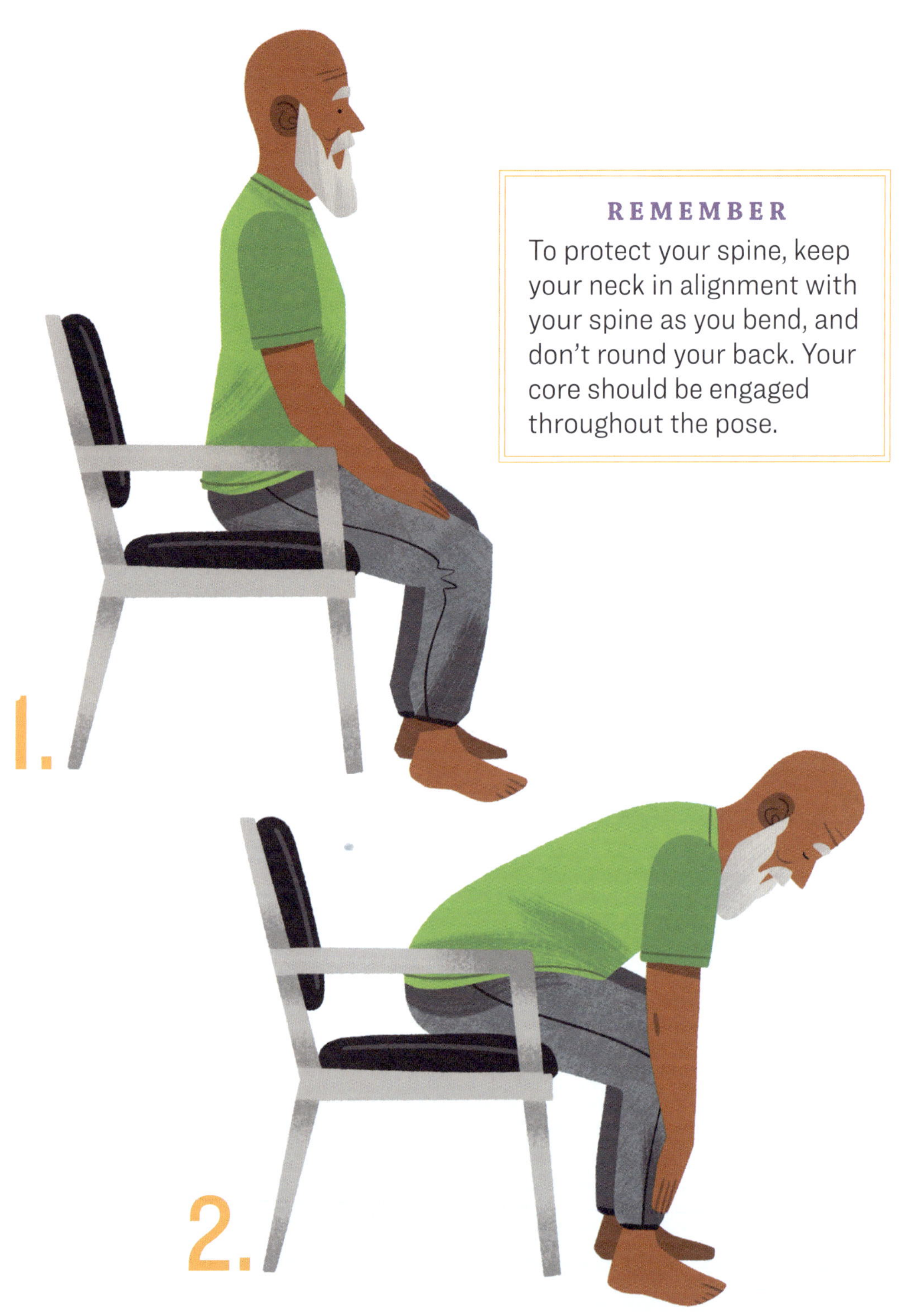


**REMEMBER**

To protect your spine, keep your neck in alignment with your spine as you bend, and don't round your back. Your core should be engaged throughout the pose.

# SEATED FORWARD FOLD

## UTTANASANA

**TARGETED AREAS:** Back, glutes, hamstrings, hip flexors, shoulders

Seated Forward Fold is a foundational pose that appears as a step in many yoga poses. It engages the entire body. The pose improves flexibility and posture, making everyday movements like bending to pick up objects or reaching for items easier and safer.

### INSTRUCTIONS

1. From Seated Mountain (page 10), inhale and bend forward gently from your hips, leading with your chest, keeping your back straight.
2. Exhale and lower your torso toward your thighs, moving your hands down your thighs and shins, reaching toward your feet or the floor, stopping at a comfortable level.
3. Take 3 to 5 rounds of breath. Come out of the pose by tapping into your core. On an inhale, lift up, keeping your spine straight as if you were being pushed up by the fronts of your shoulders.

To simplify, decrease the angle of your bend and/or place a pillow on your thighs and rest your forearms on it.

For a challenge, lift your arms, keeping them straight and aligned with your ears.

**Keep in Mind:** A full Forward Fold—in which your head is below your heart—may be dangerous for people with high blood pressure or heart issues. If you have either, check with your healthcare professional before doing this pose. An alternative is to keep the head above or level with your heart.

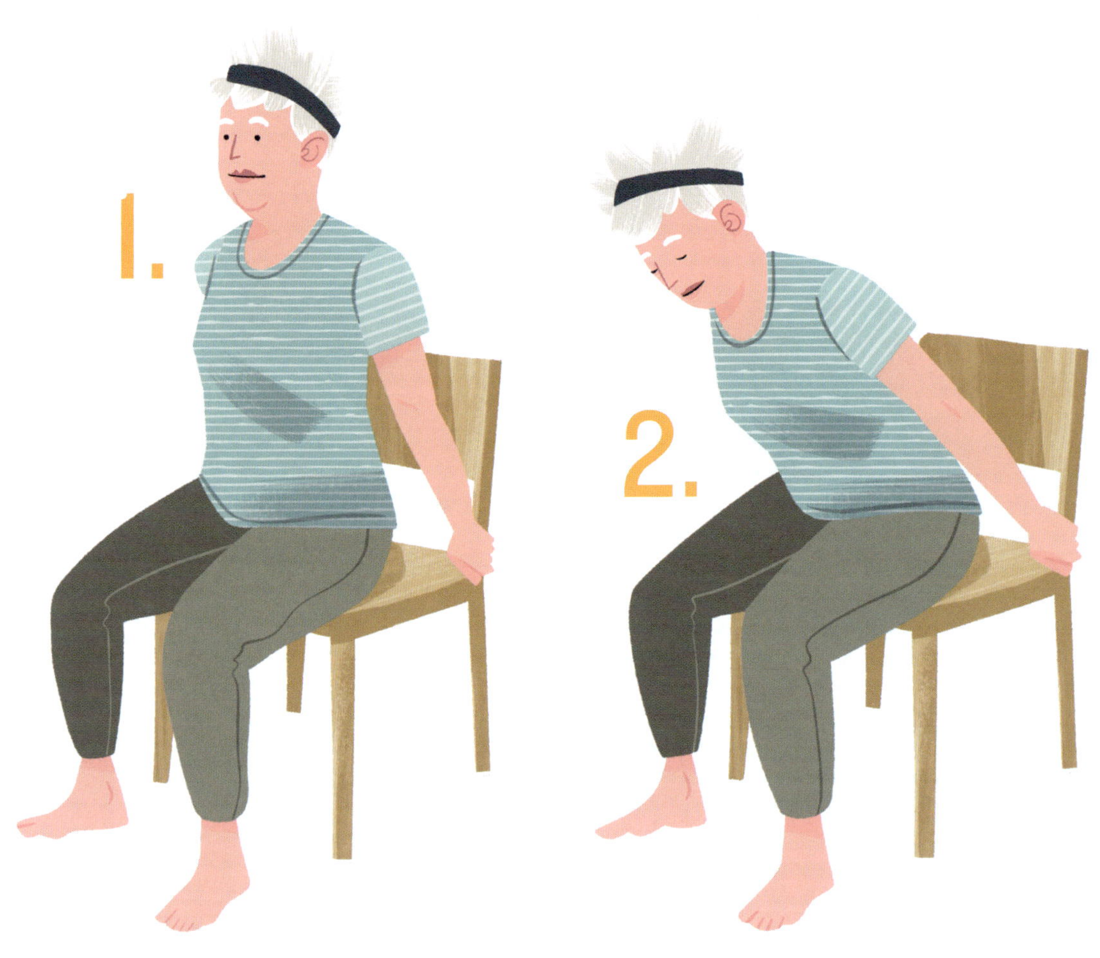


**REMEMBER**

Keep your neck in line with your spine. Relax your shoulders, keeping them down and away from your ears.

# SEATED FORWARD FOLD WITH SHOULDER STRETCH

## BADDHA HASTA UTTANASANA

**TARGETED AREAS:** Arms, back, chest, core, shoulders

This pose helps you gently stretch your back, chest, and shoulders while improving flexibility and posture. It helps with posture problems, like a hunched mid-back, and improves the flexibility of your thoracic spine. It's a great remedy to relieve tension, especially if you've been sitting for a while.

### INSTRUCTIONS

1. From Seated Mountain (page 10) inhale and gently pull your shoulders back, reaching both hands back to lightly grab the back of the chair comfortably.
2. Exhale and bend at the hips, leaning your upper body forward and keeping your back straight. Keep your chest open and your shoulder blades squeezed together behind your back. Let your torso move toward your thighs while maintaining a light grip on the chair back. Keep your elbows soft to avoid overextending. Hold the stretch for 3 to 5 rounds of breath.
3. To come out of the stretch, inhale as you tap into your core strength to gently lift your torso back to an upright seated position, releasing your grip on the chair.

To simplify, keep your arms at your sides instead of reaching back during step 1. Focus on gently opening your chest and shoulders.

For a challenge, during step 2, while leaning forward, let go of the chair and interlace your fingers behind your back. For an even deeper stretch, lift your interlaced arms upward.

**Keep in Mind:** To avoid straining your shoulders or wrists, don't pull too hard on the back of the chair. Instead, maintain a light grip and keep your elbows slightly bent to protect your joints and prevent hyperextension. To protect your back, keep your core engaged, pulling belly button to spine throughout.

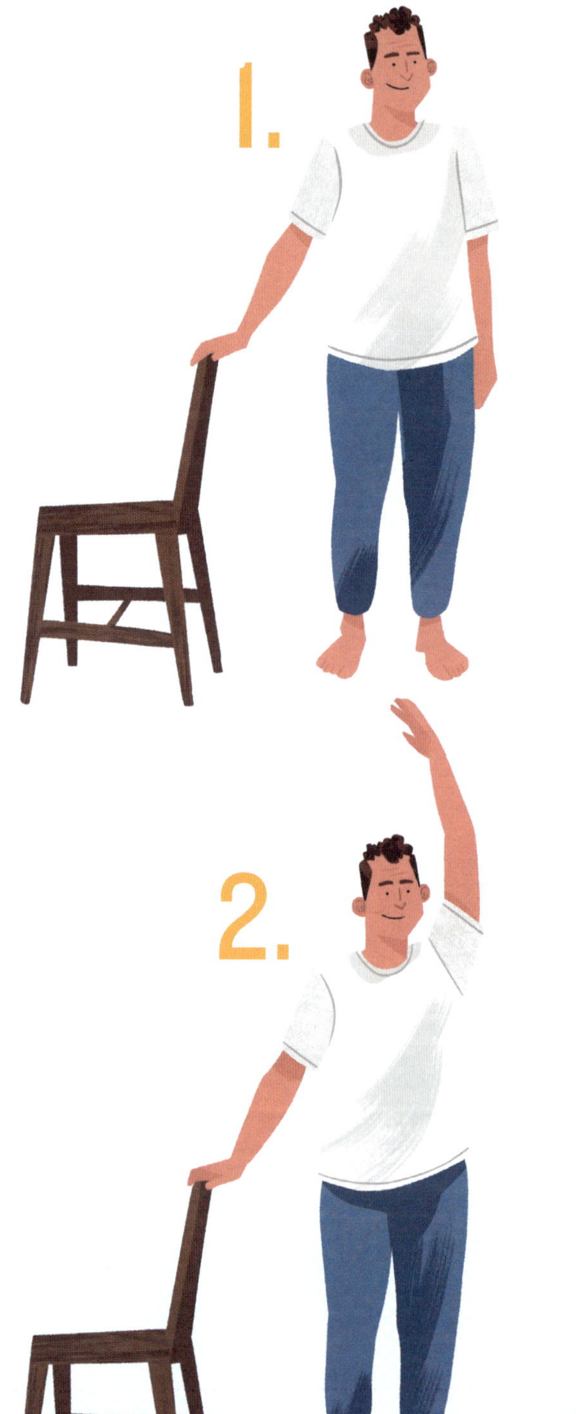


**REMEMBER**

Engage your core by pulling your belly button in toward your spine and imagine a string pulling your head up at the top to feel your body lift.

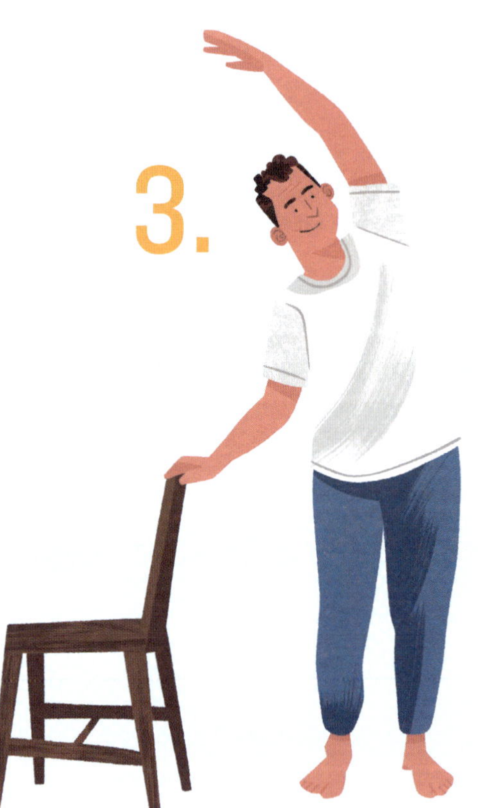

# STANDING SIDE STRETCH

## PARSVA TADASANA

**TARGETED AREAS:** Arms, chest, neck, shoulders, sides, spine, upper back

This pose is one of my favorite stretches when I've been working at the computer for hours. It reduces stiffness in my back and sides, improves my posture, and promotes better breathing by opening up the rib cage. It also strengthens the core and improves flexibility for everyday movements.

### INSTRUCTIONS

1. Stand with your feet hip-width apart, with your right side next to the back of the chair and your right hand on the back of the chair.
2. Inhale, activating your core and raising your left arm overhead, close to your ear, with a soft bend in your elbow.
3. Exhale and lean to your right, creating a stretch along the left side of your body.
4. Hold for 3 to 5 rounds of breath. Repeat on the other side.

To simplify, take a seat. Bend to the side while holding on to the side of the chair, extending the left side long as you lean to the right.

For a challenge, lift both arms and lean to one side. Palms can be kept separate or brought together in prayer position (see page 72, Seated Revolved Chair), strengthening your shoulders and arms.

**Keep in Mind:** To focus on the stretch in your torso, keep your hips still and facing forward for the entire stretch. Stay within a comfortable range of motion.

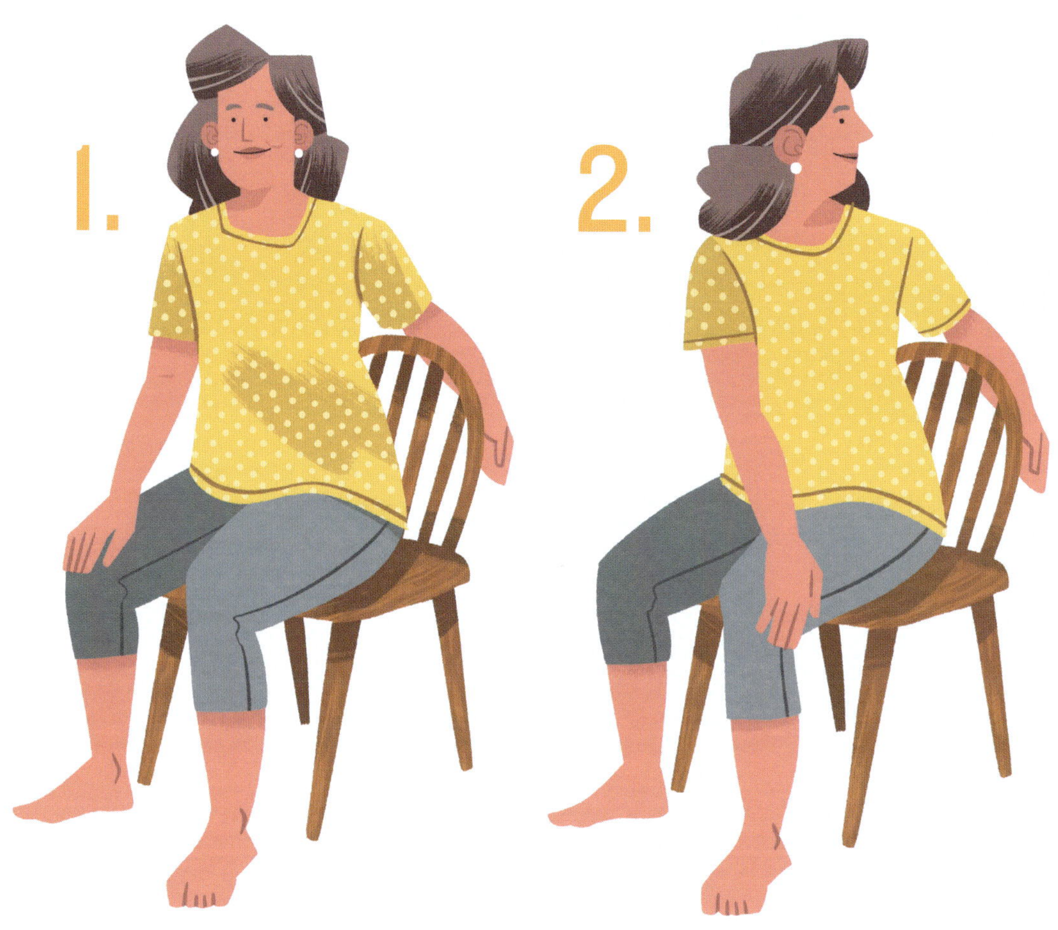


**REMEMBER**

Keep your spine lengthened throughout the twist and don't round your back. Also, make sure your knees are aligned directly over your ankles for stability.

# SEATED SPINAL TWIST

## PARIVRTTA TADASANA

**TARGETED AREAS:** Back, core, neck, spine

Being able to turn or rotate is essential for everyday tasks such as putting your seat belt on or looking over your shoulder. Seated Spinal Twist improves spine flexibility, makes rotational movements easier, and strengthens core muscles to improve posture. It can also alleviate lower back tension.

### INSTRUCTIONS

1. From Seated Mountain (page 10), inhale and place your left forearm over the back of the chair for support and place your right hand on the outside of your left thigh.
2. Exhale and gently twist your upper body to the left, leading the movement with your torso rather than pulling with your arms. Look back toward your left arm if possible. Take 3 to 5 rounds of breath. With each inhale, lengthen your spine, thinking tall. With each exhale, you may deepen the twist slightly if it feels comfortable.
3. Slowly untwist to return to the starting position. Repeat on the other side with your right forearm over the back of the chair.

To simplify, keep your left arm at your side when your right hand is on the outside of your left knee, and vice versa.

For a challenge, lift your back arm off the chair and move it back farther, engaging the torso.

**Keep in Mind:** If you have back issues or osteoporosis, consult with your healthcare professional before doing this pose. To avoid straining your spine or surrounding muscles, twist only to a natural point.

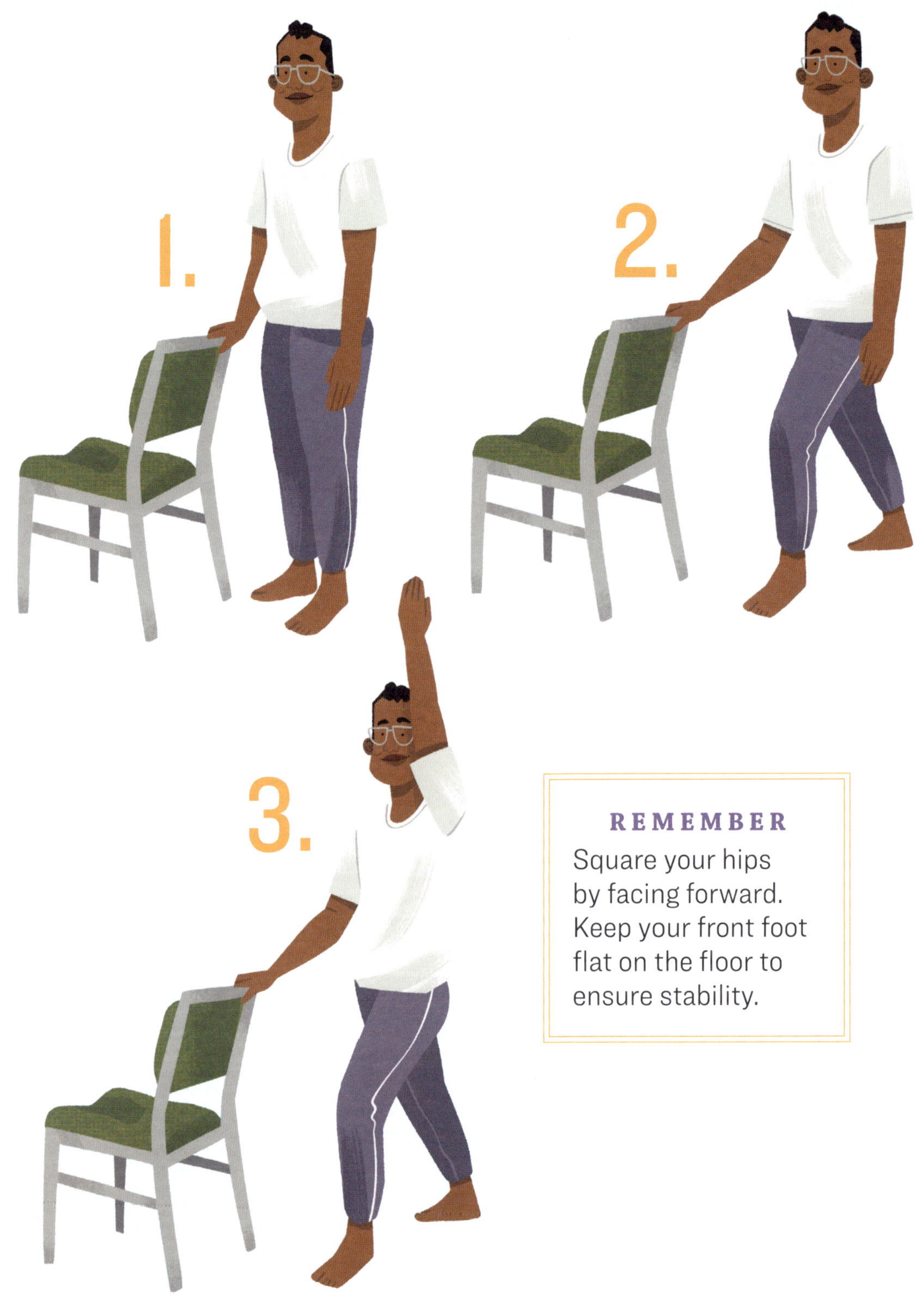


**REMEMBER**

Square your hips by facing forward. Keep your front foot flat on the floor to ensure stability.

# STANDING WARRIOR I

## VIRABHADRASANA I

**TARGETED AREAS:** Arms, back, core, hips, legs, shoulders

Sitting a lot can tighten muscles including the hip flexors, which are important for staying mobile. Warrior I improves upper- and lower-body flexibility, including opening up the hips and chest and strengthening the core.

## INSTRUCTIONS

1. Stand to the side of your chair with your right hand resting on the back of the chair.
2. Inhale and step your right foot back, grounding your toes and heel. The front left knee is bent, stacked in alignment with your ankle.
3. With your right hand on the chair for stability, exhale and lift your left arm straight overhead, palm facing inward. Keep your shoulders relaxed and away from your ears. Hold this pose for 3 to 5 rounds of breath and switch sides.

To simplify, take a seat. Sit sideways, with the left corner of the chair between your thighs. Place your left foot flat on the floor with your left knee aligned over your ankle. Extend your right leg straight back, keeping your knee slightly bent, right foot flat on floor and both heels aligned.

For a challenge, raise both arms overhead. You can also bend the front knee more as is comfortable.

**Keep in Mind:** Don't force the back leg too far back or overextend the arms if doing so causes discomfort. Keep movements smooth and controlled and listen to your body to prevent strain or injury.

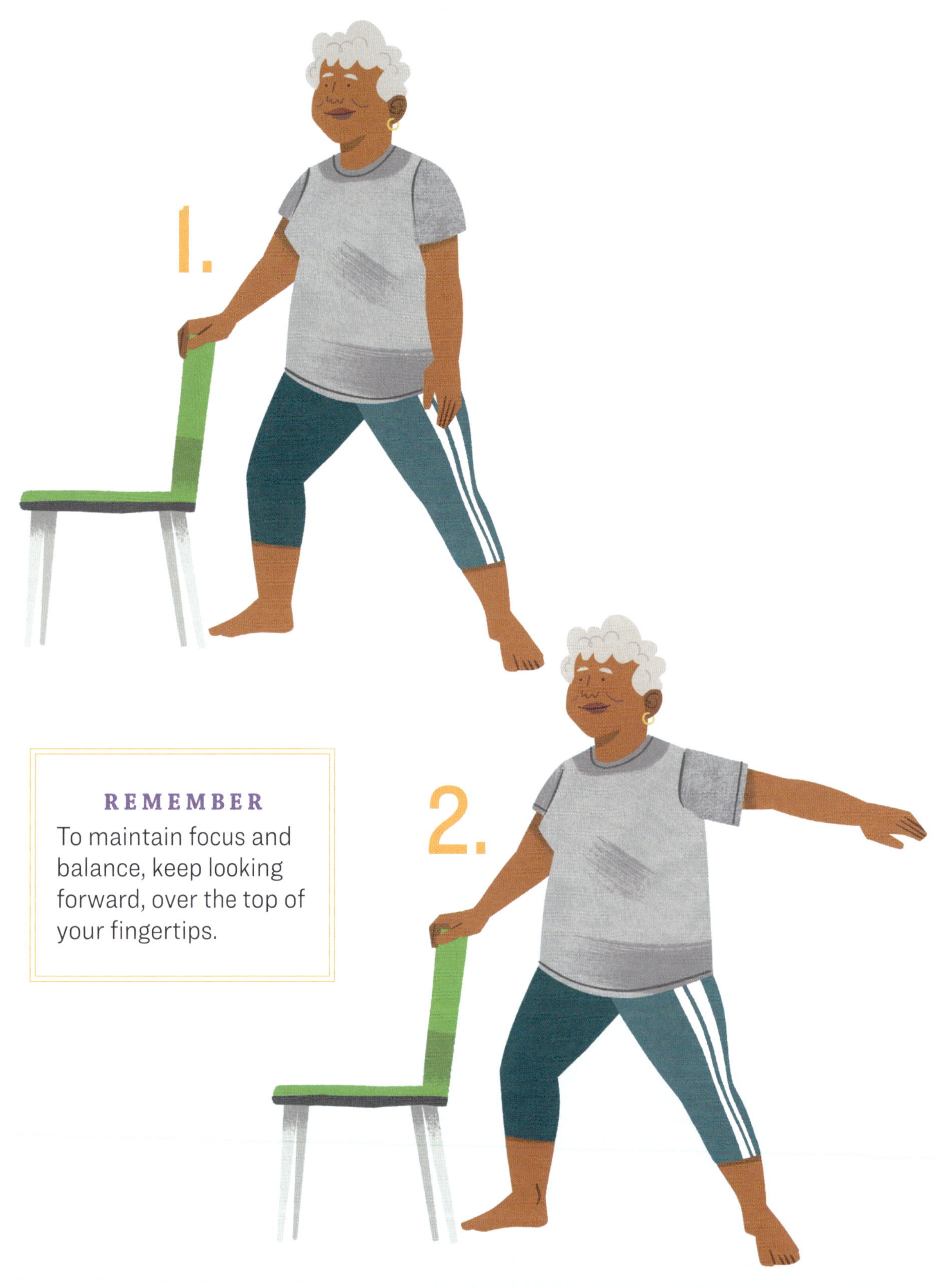


**REMEMBER**

To maintain focus and balance, keep looking forward, over the top of your fingertips.

# STANDING WARRIOR II

## VIRABHADRASANA II

**TARGETED AREAS:** Arms, core, legs, shoulders

While all of the Warrior poses build strength and flexibility in the legs, hips, and core, Warrior II's specific focus on stretching outward when the arms are extended enhances balance, improves upper-body flexibility, and opens the rib cage for better breathing. This pose requires you to stand behind your chair for stability rather than next to it. Experiment with the simplified modification if you want to build up to less chair support.

### INSTRUCTIONS

1. Stand behind your chair with room to move. Your feet should be hip-width apart for better balance and stability. Imagine both your feet are on railroad tracks that are hip-width apart. Hold on to the back of the chair with your right hand. Inhale and step your left foot back, opening up your hips, with your toes pointing away from your body. Bend your right leg with your knee over your ankle.
2. Exhale and extend your left arm to the side at shoulder level, palm facing down, reaching through your fingertips with a soft bend in your elbow. Keep your shoulder relaxed. Hold this pose for 3 to 5 rounds of breath, then switch sides.

To simplify, take a seat. Sit sideways on the chair facing left and place your left foot flat on the floor, extending your right leg back. Extend the back leg as far as is comfortable and try to put your foot flat on the floor. If this is uncomfortable, bend the back leg so that the knee is over the ankle for stability. Place your hands on your hips as in Standing Warrior I (page 36) or extend both arms out at shoulder height if comfortable.

For a challenge, extend both arms without holding on to the chair.

**Keep in Mind:** To provide a solid foundation, make sure your feet are firmly planted on the floor.

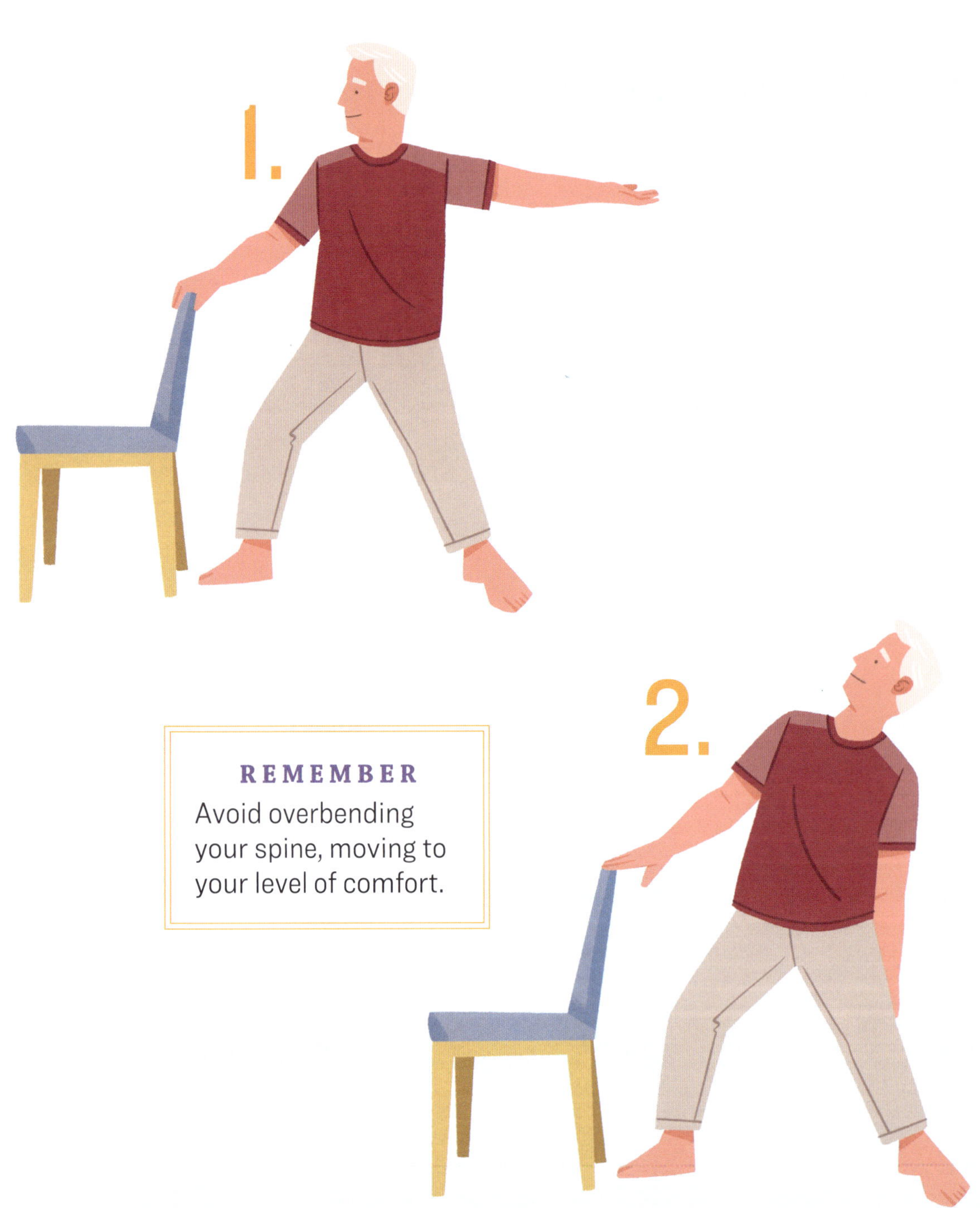


**REMEMBER**

Avoid overbending your spine, moving to your level of comfort.

# STANDING REVERSE WARRIOR

## VIPARITA VIRABHADRASANA

**TARGETED AREAS:** Arms, back/spine, core, legs, shoulders

The positioning of Standing Reverse Warrior starts with Warrior II. Like that pose, it strengthens your legs and core and improves balance. Unlike Warrior II's focus on static alignment and balance, Reverse Warrior emphasizes lengthening the side body and spine.

### INSTRUCTIONS

1. Begin in Standing Warrior II (page 39), with your back left foot turned inward for comfort. Inhale and turn your palm up on your extended left arm.
2. Exhale and sweep your left arm overhead and slightly back, reaching toward the ceiling or slightly behind you. Relax your shoulder down your back, and keep your core engaged. Look up at your raised hand or keep your gaze forward for comfort.
3. Take 3 rounds of breath, then switch sides and repeat the sequence.

To simplify, take a seat. From Seated Warrior II, allow the back arm to gently slide down your back leg for support. If extending your arms is difficult, rest your front arm on your thigh and back hand on your hip.

For a challenge, reach toward the floor with your back arm to engage your back and shoulders.

**Keep in Mind:** Don't overextend your spine. Keep the movement gentle and within your comfortable range of motion to prevent strain in your neck and lower back.

**REMEMBER**

Keep your spine long and upright to enhance the stretch and improve posture.

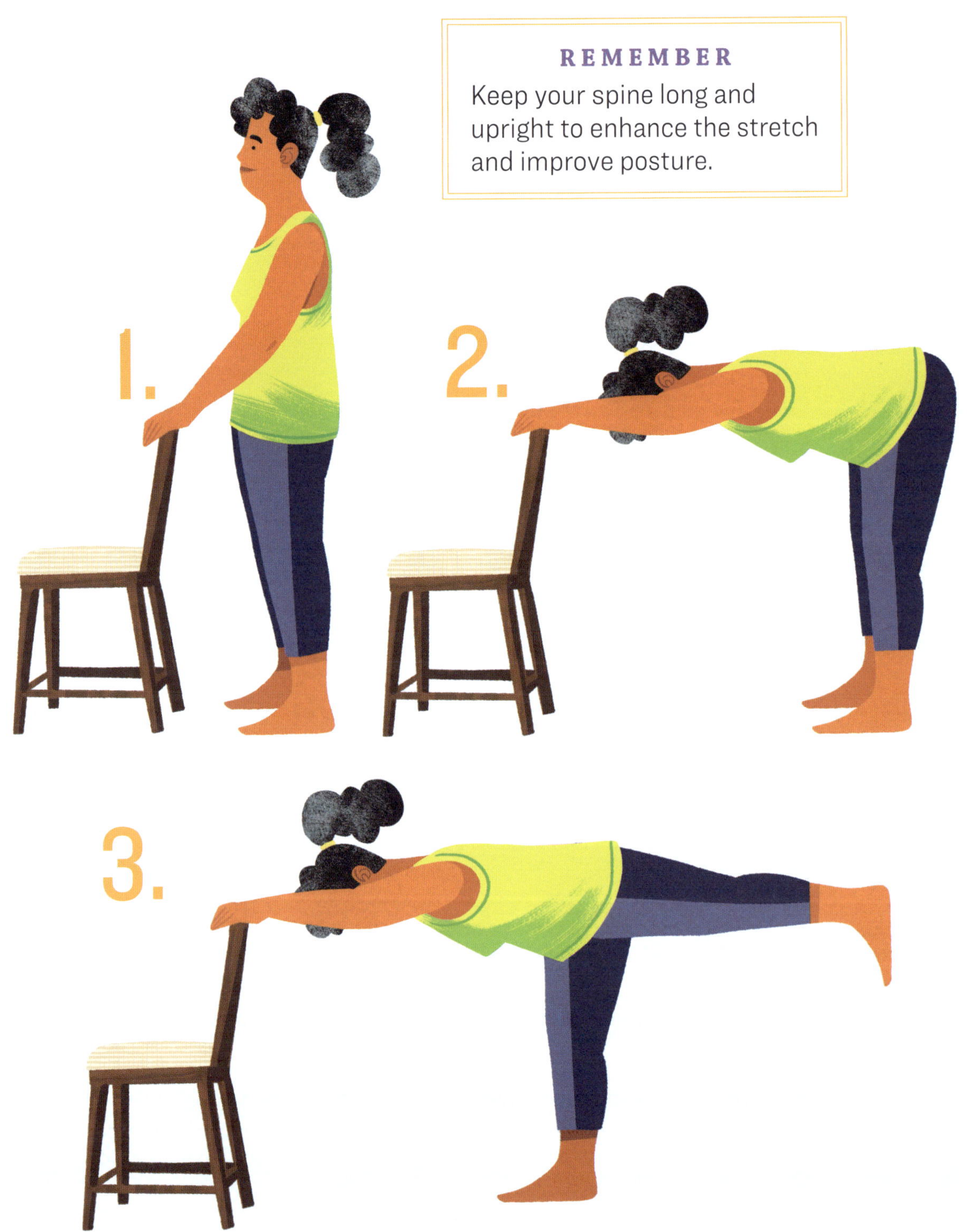

# STANDING WARRIOR III

## VIRABHADRASANA III

**TARGETED AREAS:** Arms, back, core, feet, glutes, hips, shoulders

This powerful pose strengthens the legs and increases upper-body flexibility in the shoulders, back, and arms. It improves balance and posture, both of which make everyday activities easier and help prevent falls. Your quads and glutes benefit from the lifted leg that distinguishes this pose from Standing Warrior I.

## INSTRUCTIONS

1. Stand facing the back of the chair with your feet hip-width apart and grip the top of the chair lightly with both hands. Begin engaging your core to avoid rounding your back.
2. Inhale, step back from the chair, and bend at the hips until your arms and back are straight and parallel to the floor. Make sure to push down and not pull the chair toward you, making it tip over.
3. Softly bending your knees, lift your left leg back and up, heel toward the ceiling, toe slightly flexed. Aim to form a straight line with your body, aligning your leg with your back, arms, and neck. Hold for 3 to 5 rounds of breath and switch sides.

To simplify, lift just your heel off the floor, pointing toes, or lift your foot only slightly.

For a challenge, when lifting the left leg, lift your right arm above the chair, parallel to the floor.

**Keep in Mind:** To protect your back, keep your hips square, with the front of your body facing the floor. Do not turn your torso.

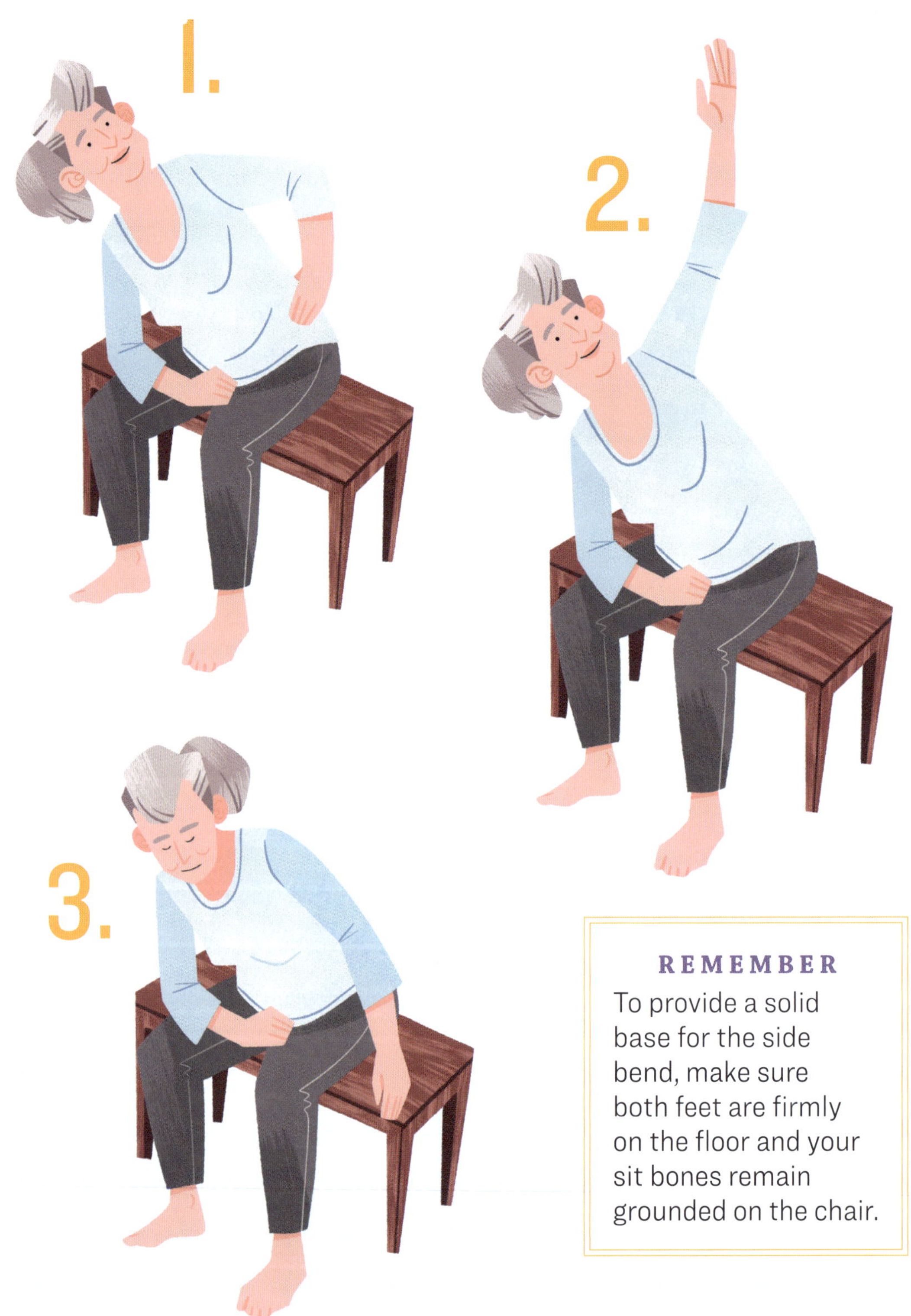


**REMEMBER**

To provide a solid base for the side bend, make sure both feet are firmly on the floor and your sit bones remain grounded on the chair.

# SEATED EXTENDED SIDE ANGLE

## UTTHITA PARSVAKONASANA

**TARGETED AREAS:** Arms, back, core

Everyday tasks like gardening or cleaning your home require ease of rotational and twisting movement. Seated Extended Side Angle enhances your range of motion, promotes better posture, and builds stability in your back and core.

### INSTRUCTIONS

1. From Seated Mountain (page 10), inhale and lay your right forearm on your thigh about 2 inches above your right knee, keeping your chest open and spine lengthened.
2. Exhale as you extend your left arm overhead, palm facing forward, opening up your chest muscles. Aim to create a long line from your left hip through your fingertips. Keep your gaze forward, or, if doing so is comfortable, look up toward your extended arm. Hold the pose, focusing on deepening the reach. Take 3 rounds of breath.
3. Return to the starting position on an inhale, sitting upright and bringing your arm back down. Repeat on the other side, placing your left elbow on your left thigh and extending your right arm overhead.

To simplify, place your left hand on your hip instead of extending it up.

For a challenge, in step 1, straighten your arm and let your palm come to meet the outside of your calf, hovering over the floor.

**Keep in Mind:** The side bend begins by sitting tall and lengthening your spine to prevent slouching. Keep your back straight and then tilt gently to the side.

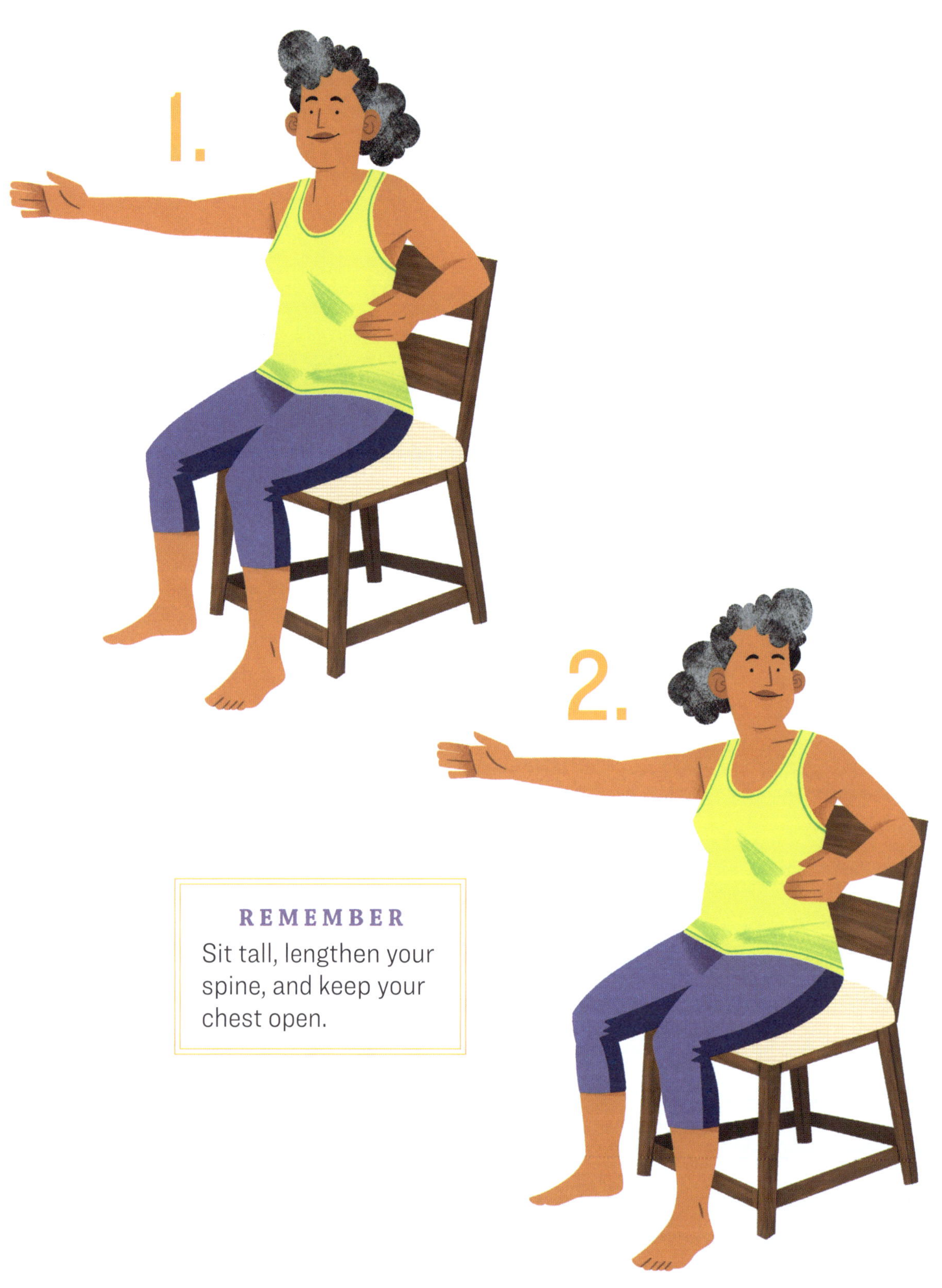


**REMEMBER**

Sit tall, lengthen your spine, and keep your chest open.

# SEATED ARCHER

## AKARNA DHANURASANA

**TARGETED AREAS:** Core, neck, shoulders, upper back

You'll feel powerful with Seated Archer, which targets upper-body flexibility, which provides numerous benefits for daily life, including improved posture and greater mobility for basic movements like checking behind you as you back out of a parking spot. Extending the arm in front of you increases strength and shoulder stability to help you lift things overhead.

### INSTRUCTIONS

1. From Seated Mountain (page 10), inhale and extend your right arm straight in front of you at shoulder height, keeping your palm facing inward as if holding a bow.
2. Bend your left elbow 90 degrees at your side, curling your fingers or making a fist.
3. Exhale and pull your left elbow back as though drawing a bowstring. Keep your gaze forward for neck comfort, or follow your back arm with your eyes, turning your head, to gently stretch your neck.
4. Take 3 to 5 rounds of breath, then switch sides.

To simplify, let your right hand rest on your knee rather than raising it. Straighten your arm to feel your arm engage.

For a challenge, turn your torso to move the pulled left arm farther back and lift your opposite right foot an inch off the ground to engage your core.

**Keep in Mind:** If you have osteoporosis, consult with your healthcare professional before trying this pose. Do not twist if you experience spinal discomfort; instead, skip step 3.

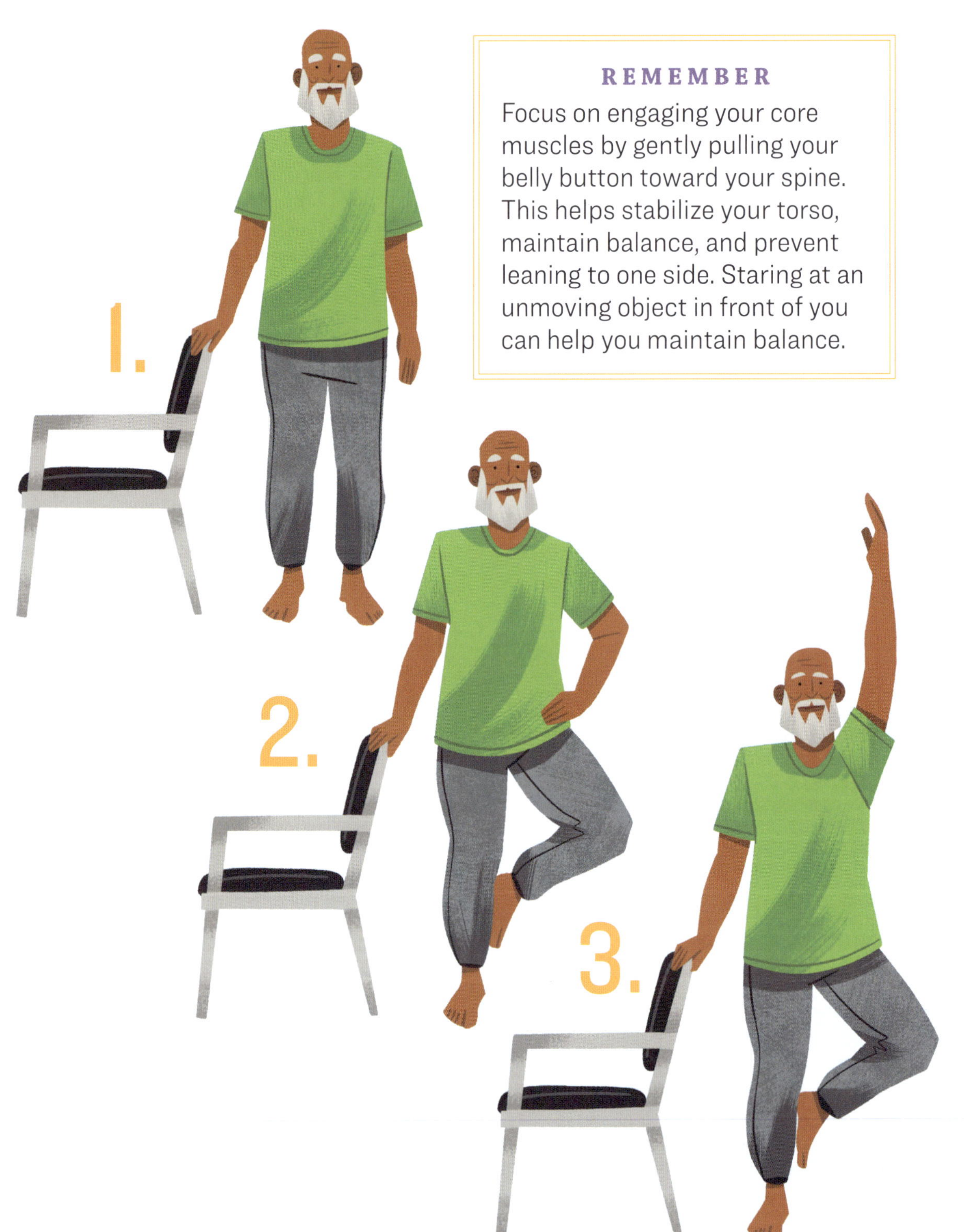


**REMEMBER**

Focus on engaging your core muscles by gently pulling your belly button toward your spine. This helps stabilize your torso, maintain balance, and prevent leaning to one side. Staring at an unmoving object in front of you can help you maintain balance.

# STANDING TREE POSE

## VRKSASANA

**TARGETED AREAS:** Arms, core, feet, hips, legs, shoulders, thighs

By training the body to stabilize itself while shifting weight and standing on one leg, Standing Tree creates a solid foundation for improving balance and stability. This single-leg move strengthens your ability to walk, climb stairs, and get into and out of the bathtub with confidence.

## INSTRUCTIONS

1. Stand sideways at the back of the chair with feet hip-width apart and your right hand on the back of the chair for stability. You can put your left hand at your side or on your hip. Your right foot can face forward or slightly turned out for comfort.
2. Inhale, placing the sole of your left foot on the inside of your right calf below your knee, creating a triangle shape with your leg. Exhale, focusing on pointing your left knee out to your left side, opening up your left hip.
3. Your left hand can sweep up overhead or stay at your side or on your hip. Take 3 rounds of breath and repeat on the other side.

To simplify, keep your feet hip-width apart, place your heel above the inside of your left ankle, and keep your toes on the ground while opening your right knee outward.

For a challenge, raise one or both arms overhead, or use your hands to place the sole of your left foot on the inside of your right thigh.

**Keep in Mind:** Keep your supporting foot firmly on the floor. Do not place the sole of your foot on your knee or ankle joint.

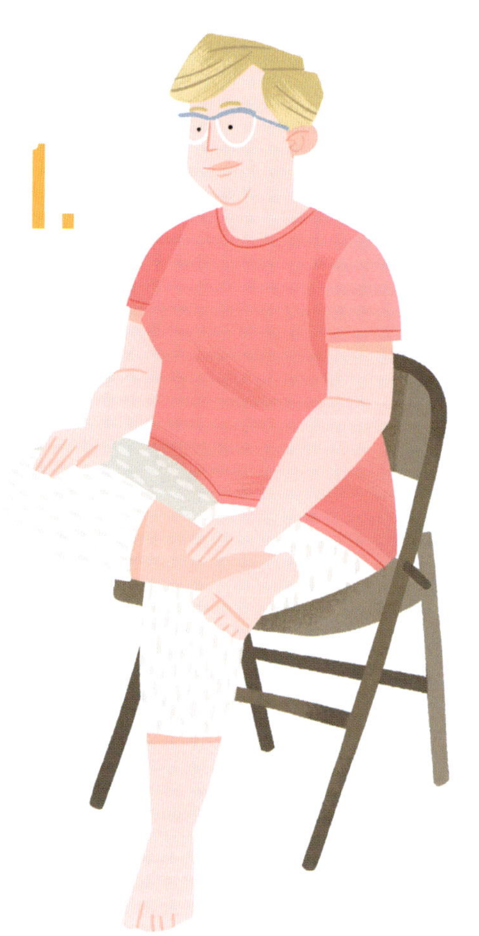


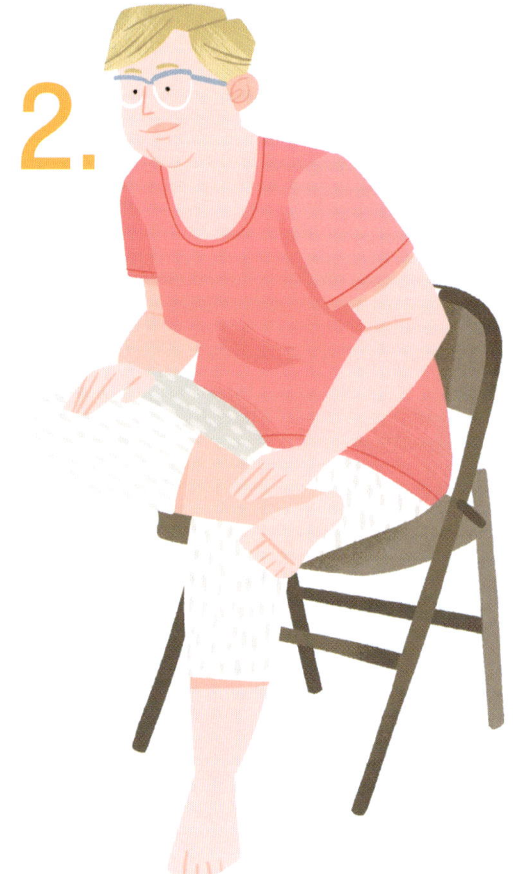


**REMEMBER**

Protect your spine by keeping your back straight and not rounding your shoulders.

# SEATED PIGEON

## KAPOTASANA

**TARGETED AREAS:** Glutes, hips, lower back

Seated Pigeon gently opens up the hips and can counterbalance the effects of sitting for long periods. This pose will support the all-important hip joints in helping you carry yourself with assurance and make other poses, from Seated Horse (page 60) to Standing Warrior III (page 42), that much more rewarding.

### INSTRUCTIONS

1. From Seated Mountain (page 10), inhale and cross your right ankle over your left thigh, creating a "figure 4" shape with your legs. You will feel the stretch in the inner hip and glute. Let your hands rest comfortably on your hips or on your lap.
2. Exhale, bending at your hips, keeping your back straight. Flex your right foot, and with your right hand above your right knee, gently press your right inner thigh down for a light stretch.
3. Take 3 to 5 rounds of breath. Repeat on the other side.

To simplify, cross your right ankle over your left ankle instead of your left thigh. Skip leaning forward if the pose is already intense.

For a challenge, gently press your right inner thigh down with your right hand above, and not on, your knee. For a variation that engages your core, lift your left foot off the floor and hold for 3 to 5 rounds of breath.

**Keep in Mind:** Sit evenly on the chair throughout the stretch. To avoid straining your lower back or hips, don't lean to one side.

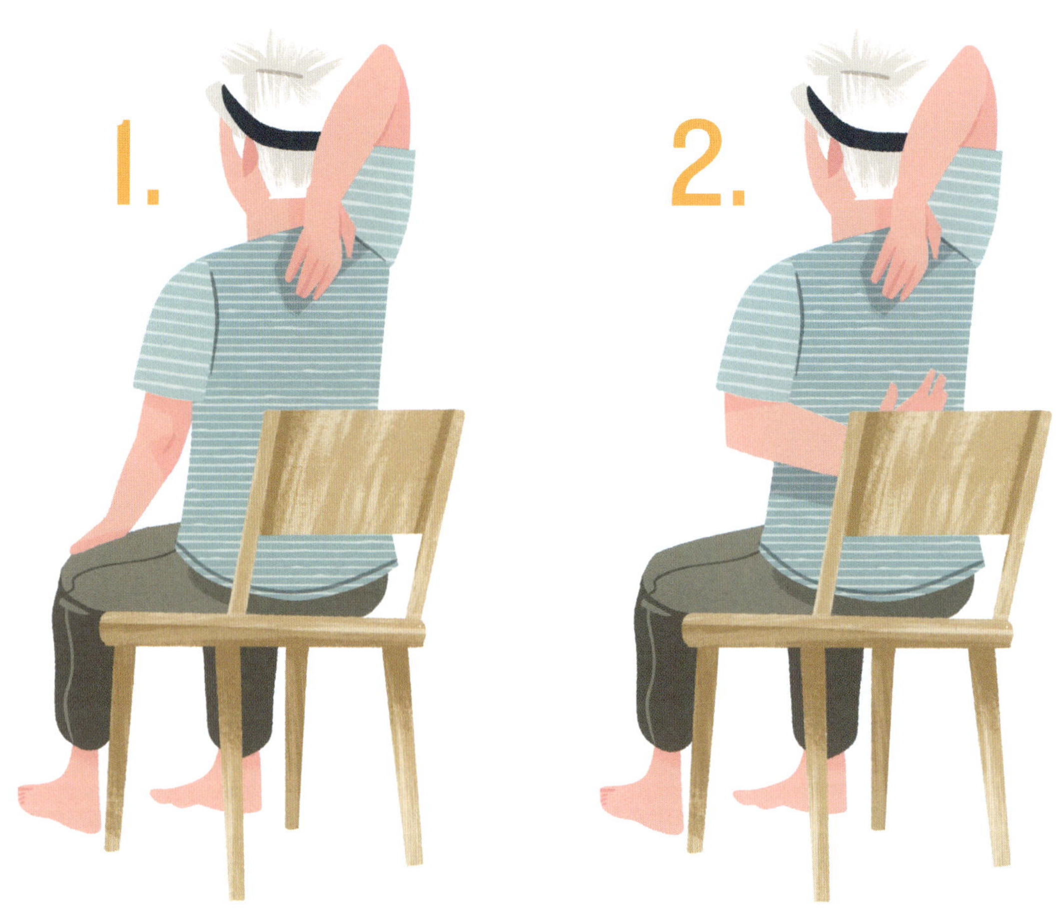


**REMEMBER**

Keep your head up and back and resist the temptation to drop your chin to your chest.

# SEATED COW FACE

## GOMUKHASANA

**TARGETED AREAS:** Arms, chest, shoulders, spine, upper back

Greater range of motion in the shoulders and arms is important for daily tasks like putting on a pullover or reaching a high shelf. Seated Cow Face strengthens posture-supporting muscles, boosts arm mobility, and improves blood flow to ease stiffness in the shoulders and upper back.

### INSTRUCTIONS

1. Inhale and raise your right arm upward, keeping your arm close to your ear with a slight bend in your elbow. Bend your elbow so your hand reaches down toward the middle of your back between your shoulder blades.
2. Exhale and gently sink a little more into the stretch. Hold the position for 3 to 5 rounds of breath and switch sides. You will feel the stretch in your shoulder joint and on the back of your upper arm.

To simplify, place your right fingers on your right shoulder and lift your elbow out to the side at a comfortable level.

For a challenge, after step 1, place the back of your left forearm on your back at waist level. Gently explore the stretch with the goal of touching the two hands together or clasping them. Take your time going into and exiting the pose.

**Keep in Mind:** If you have shoulder issues, work on exploring range of movement from the simplified modification.

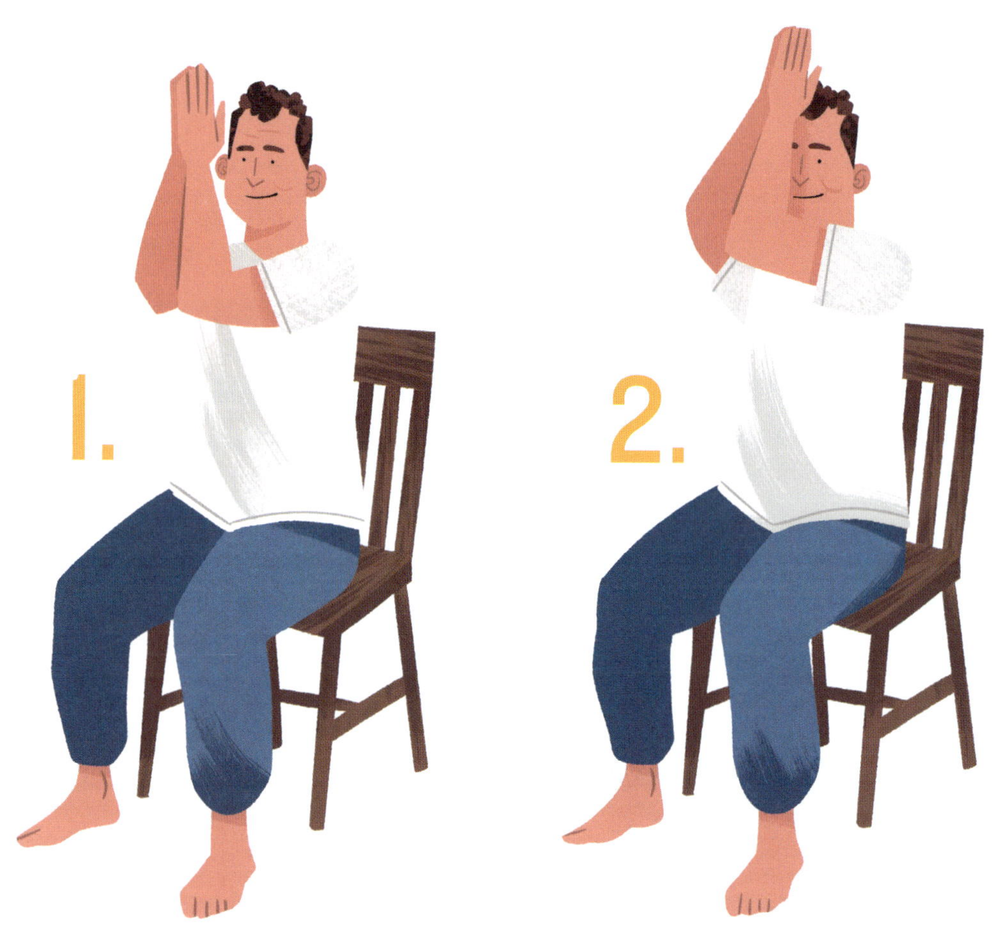


**REMEMBER**

Keep your movements gentle, avoiding any forceful pressing into the stretch.

# SEATED DOLPHIN

## ARDHA PINCHA MAYURASANA

**TARGETED AREAS:** Arms, chest, neck, shoulders, upper back

You'll be able to stand up straighter with the posture-improving Seated Dolphin. Strengthen your upper arms, increase shoulder and upper-back mobility, and reduce tension. You'll see the payoff whether you're playing racquet sports, mowing the lawn, or standing up taller in a group photo.

### INSTRUCTIONS

1. Starting in Seated Mountain (page 10), inhale and place your palms together in front of your face, aiming to put your forearms together so your elbows touch. If this is too challenging, just place your palms together and bring your elbows as close to each other as possible.
2. Exhale and gently lift your arms so your thumbs reach above your forehead. Gently squeeze your elbows together, even if they aren't touching, to engage your arms and chest.
3. Hold the pose and take 3 to 5 rounds of breath.

To simplify, place your hands on opposite shoulders, giving yourself a hug, moving your elbows as close together as possible, changing which arm is on top each time.

For a challenge, lift one foot off the floor to engage and strengthen your core.

**Keep in Mind:** To make the pose more comfortable, you can lower your arms or keep your arms and palms apart during the pose.

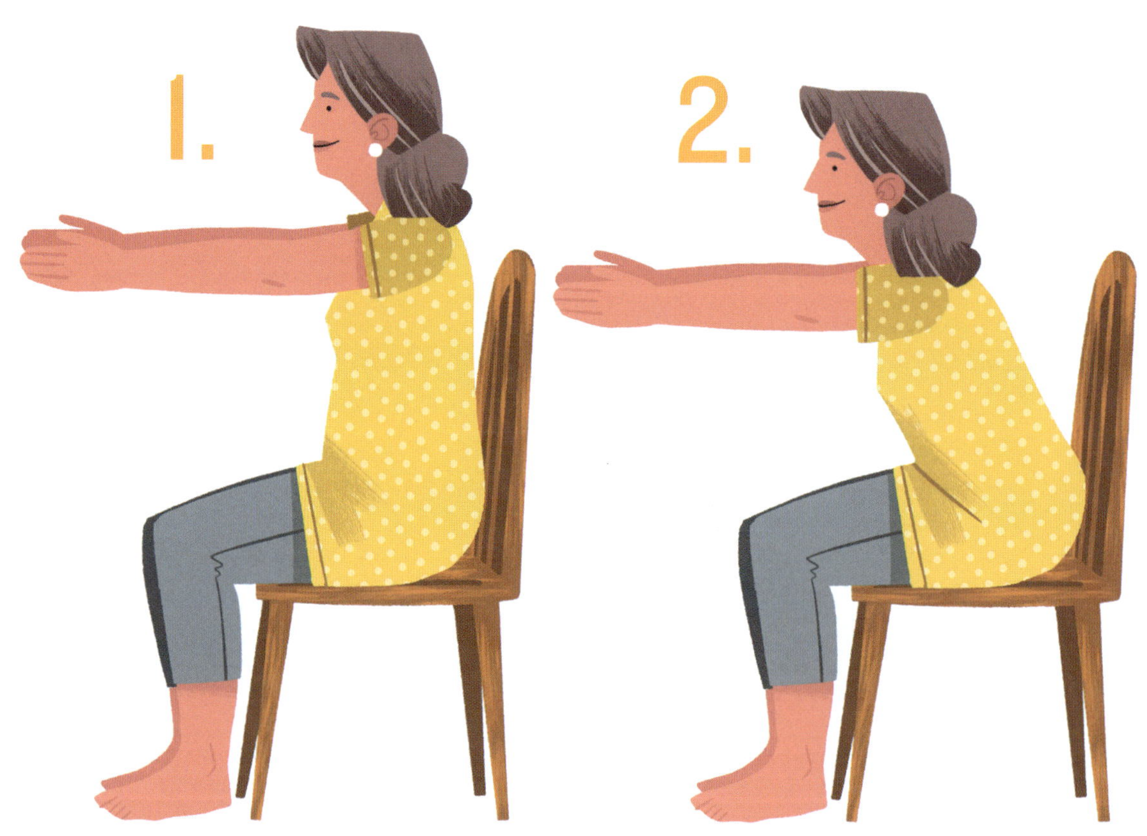


**REMEMBER**

Align your knees above your ankles, keep your back straight, press your feet firmly into the floor, and relax your shoulders.

# SEATED CHAIR

## UTKATASANA

**TARGETED AREAS:** Full body (arms, back, core, feet/ankles, glutes, legs, shoulders)

This is the all-in-one pose with the perfect name—let's be the chair! While similar to the Seated Mountain from which the pose begins, Seated Chair targets the activation of the core and legs, while Seated Mountain helps you become accustomed to the alignment necessary for attaining chair yoga's benefits.

### INSTRUCTIONS

1. From Seated Mountain (page 10), inhale and pull your belly button gently toward your spine to engage your core muscles and lengthen your spine. Imagine a string is pulling you up from the top of your head. Raise your arms forward to shoulder height, palms facing inward.
2. Exhale and press your feet firmly into the ground as if trying to lift yourself slightly off the chair. Feel your thighs and glutes engage. Bend at the hips, keeping your back straight.
3. Hold the position and take 3 to 5 rounds of breath.

To simplify, raise your arms only as high as you can or keep them on your thighs. You can also sit upright, rather than bend forward.

For a challenge, raise your arms overhead and/or lift your butt off the chair an inch or two and hover for one to two rounds of breath, with only the back of your thighs touching the chair.

**Keep in Mind:** If you feel unsteady or notice discomfort in your knees, reduce the depth of the pose by sitting farther back in the chair for added support.

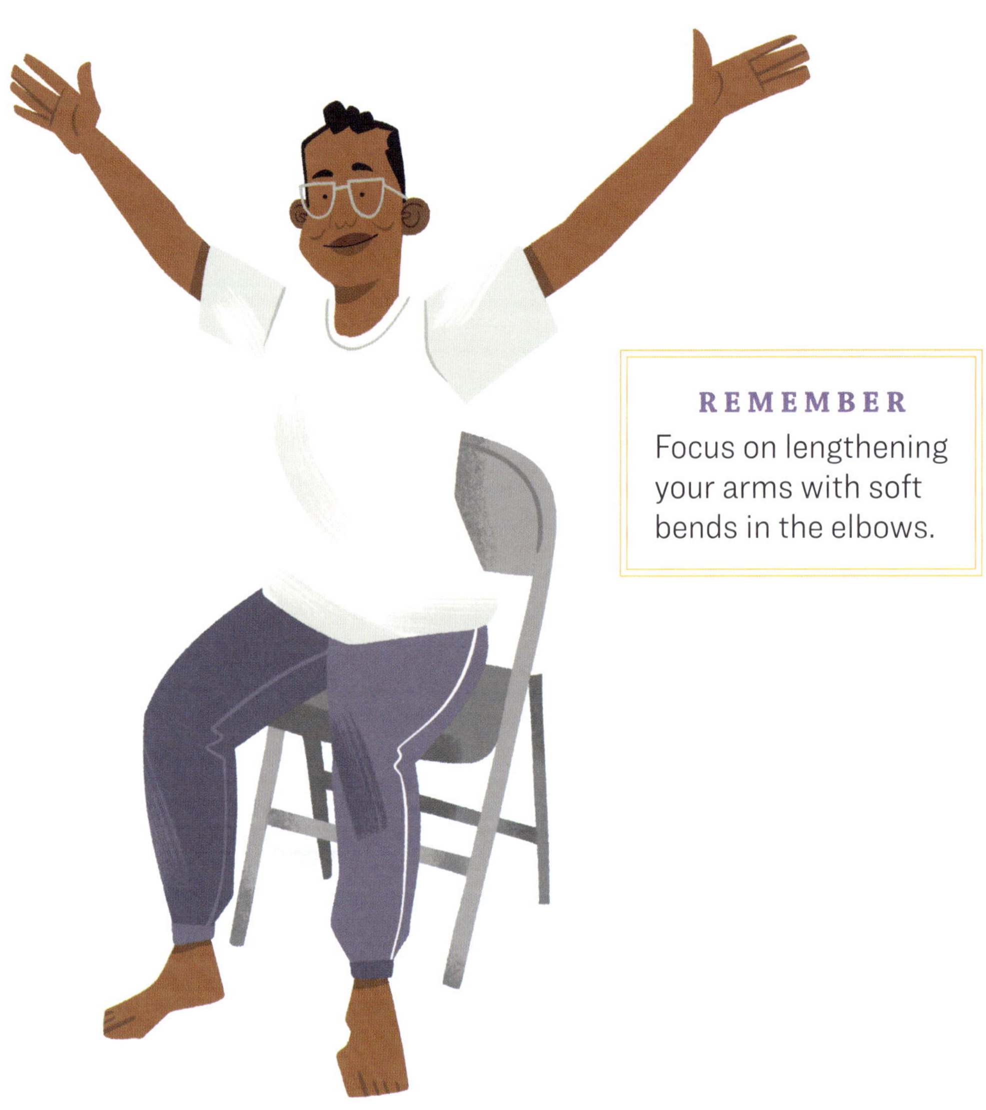

**REMEMBER**
Focus on lengthening your arms with soft bends in the elbows.

# SEATED STAR

## UTTHITA TADASANA

**TARGETED AREAS:** Arms, back, chest, shoulders

Seated Star will make you a star inside and out! This uplifting stretch opens up your chest, which improves posture and allows for deeper, more effective breathing. The upper-body expansion will allow you more range for bringing in your loved ones for big hugs, showing off all the angles of a new outfit, or reaching for a wrench while you work on a repair.

## INSTRUCTIONS

1. From Seated Mountain (page 10), exhale and pull your shoulders back, down, and away from your ears, feeling your shoulder blades move down and squeeze together behind your back. Inhale and extend your arms up diagonally in a Y-shape, palms facing forward. Spread your fingers wide, as if reaching outward to create a star shape.
2. Lift your chest slightly, lengthening through your spine and neck. Gaze forward or slightly upward. Stay in the pose for 3 to 5 rounds of breath, focusing on the stretch and the openness in your chest and shoulders.

To simplify, lower your arms to shoulder level or below.

For a challenge, alternate lifting your right and left knees, holding each lift for two to three seconds.

**Keep in Mind:** While lifting your chest, focus on lengthening your spine rather than leaning back or arching excessively. Keep your core gently engaged to support your lower back and prevent strain.

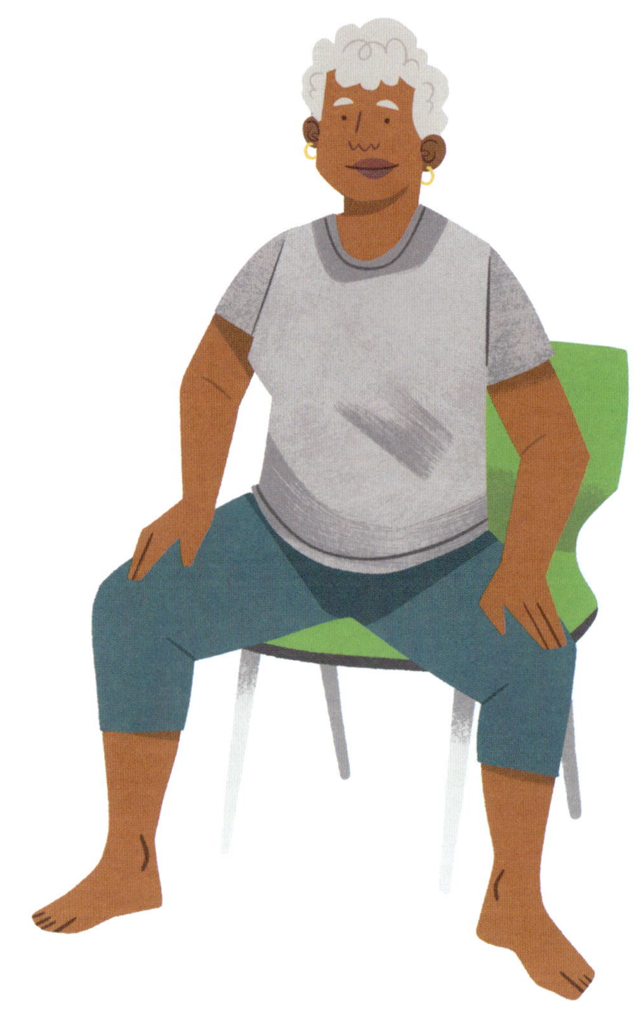

**REMEMBER**

Sit tall with a neutral spine. Pull your belly button gently toward your spine to activate your core.

# SEATED HORSE

## VATAYANASANA

**TARGETED AREAS:** Core, glutes, hips, lower back, thighs

Giddy up and stretch! The wide-legged stance of Seated Horse stretches and opens the hip joints to reduce stiffness and improve circulation. Engaging the inner thighs, core, and glutes can improve stability and balance to prevent falls and make evening walks around the neighborhood more pleasant.

## INSTRUCTIONS

1. From Seated Mountain (page 10), sit slightly forward on the chair to provide more mobility for your hips. Place your feet wider than shoulder-width apart. Point your toes out 45 degrees. Your knees should align with your ankles to create a stable base. Inhale and place your hands on your thighs or hips.
2. Keeping your back straight, exhale and press down through your feet, feeling your thighs activate. If able, activate the outsides of your hips to gently open up your knees wider.
3. Take 3 to 5 rounds of breath.

To simplify, decrease the width of your stance.

For a challenge, lean forward slightly to deepen the stretch and/or raise your heels, activating the calf muscles. Or you can lift off the chair an inch or two to hover for one to three rounds of breath.

**Keep in Mind:** To maintain stability and avoid stressing your knee joints, don't let your knees collapse inward.

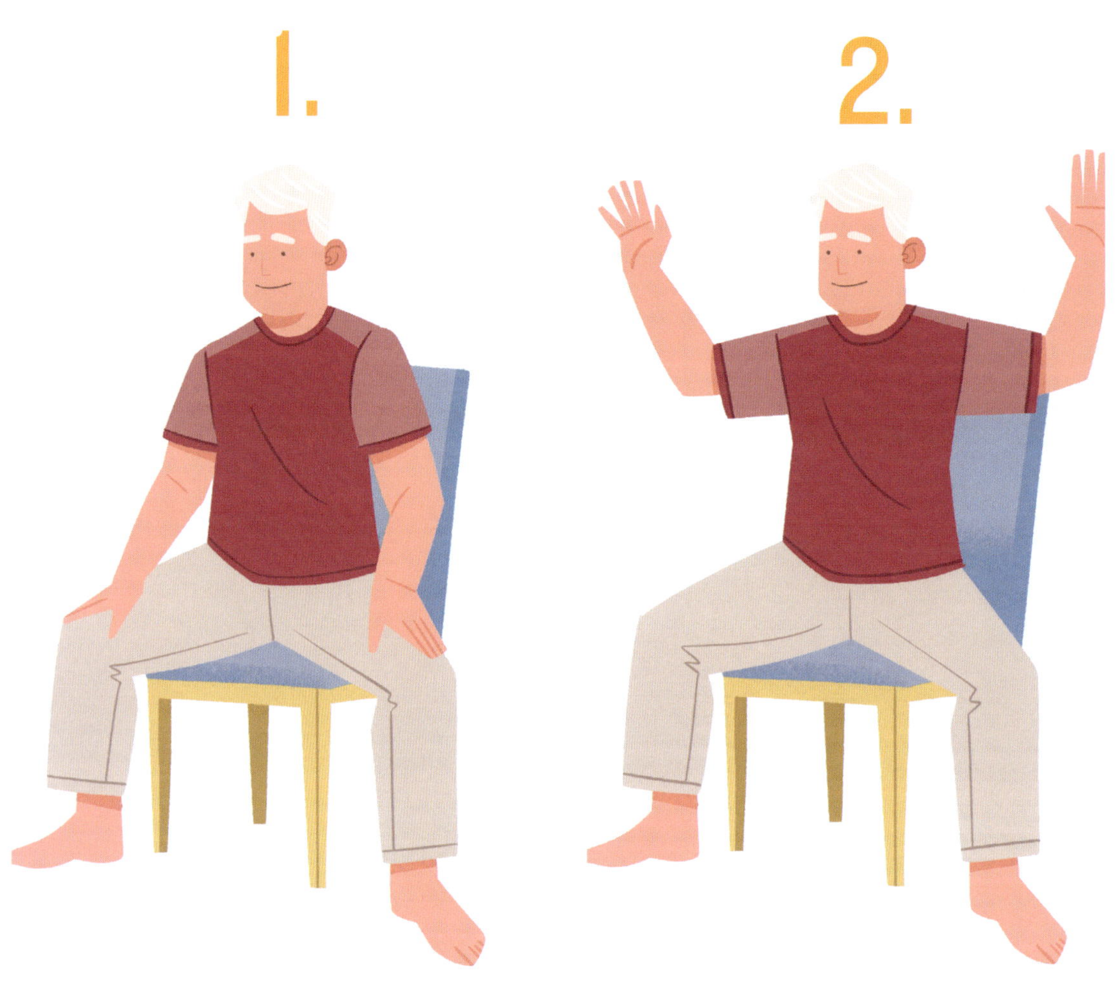


**REMEMBER**

To provide stability for the pose, press your feet into the floor to engage your thighs and hips.

# SEATED GODDESS

## UTKATA KONASANA

**TARGETED AREAS:** Arm, core, hips, shoulders, thighs

Build the strength of a goddess with this elegant pose that works the hips, thighs, and core while improving flexibility and posture. Holding the open-arm position builds shoulder and arm strength, making actions such as carrying a laundry basket easier.

## INSTRUCTIONS

1. Start in Seated Horse (page 60).
2. Inhale and bring your arms up to shoulder height, bending the elbows at a 90-degree angle so your palms face forward, forming a "cactus" shape with your arms. Exhale, engaging your core and lengthening through the spine, squeezing your shoulder blades behind your back, and keeping your chest open.
3. Take 3 to 5 rounds of breath, relaxing your shoulders away from your ears. Focus on keeping your knees pushing away from each other and pressing your feet into the floor

To simplify, lower your arms below shoulder level as in Seated Star (page 58).

For a challenge, in step 2 gently lean your upper body to one side, keeping your core engaged and spine long to increase strength and flexibility in the torso.

**Keep in Mind:** Make sure your knees remain directly over your ankles, not caving in or extending beyond your toes. This alignment protects your knee joints and ensures stability. If you feel any discomfort in your knees, reduce the angle of your toes or bring your feet closer together.

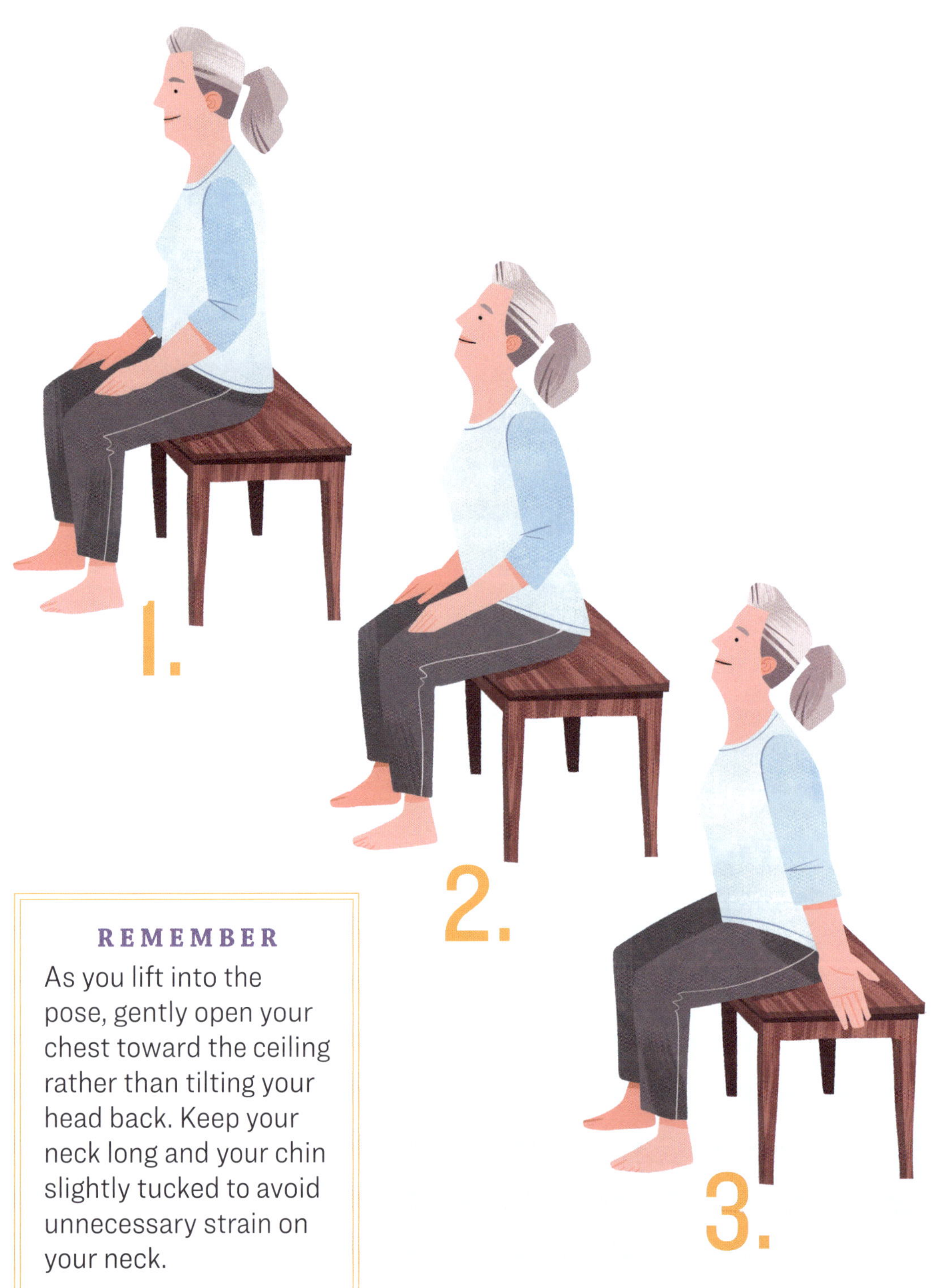


**REMEMBER**

As you lift into the pose, gently open your chest toward the ceiling rather than tilting your head back. Keep your neck long and your chin slightly tucked to avoid unnecessary strain on your neck.

# SEATED COBRA

## BHUJANGASANA

**TARGETED AREAS:** Back, chest, shoulders, spine

Strike a majestic pose with Seated Cobra! If you find yourself with neck and back tension from leaning or hunching, take a few moments to proactively counteract it with this uplifting pose. Over time, the upper-body expansion and core integrity can lead to improved posture. Let the energy moving along your spine bring a brightness to your day.

### INSTRUCTIONS

1. From "Cow" of Seated Cat-Cow (page 14), place your hands on the sides of the chair seat or on your thighs for support.
2. Roll your shoulders back and down, away from your ears, to open your chest. Imagine your collarbones gently spreading apart. Inhale deeply, lengthening your spine as you gently arch your upper back.
3. Exhale as you lift your chest toward the ceiling, keeping your shoulders relaxed and elbows slightly bent. Keep your gaze above your sight line.
4. Take 3 to 5 rounds of breath, focusing on lengthening your spine and creating space between your vertebrae.

For a challenge, as you lift your chest, lift your arms at your sides up to a forty-five-degree angle, pulling them slightly back, and spread your fingers with your palms facing forward, further stretching and strengthening the shoulders, back, and core.

**Keep in Mind:** While gazing slightly upward, avoid overextending your neck. This pose can be done in a more casual seated environment, like the sofa.

**REMEMBER**

Keep a soft bend in your extended knee to protect the joint.

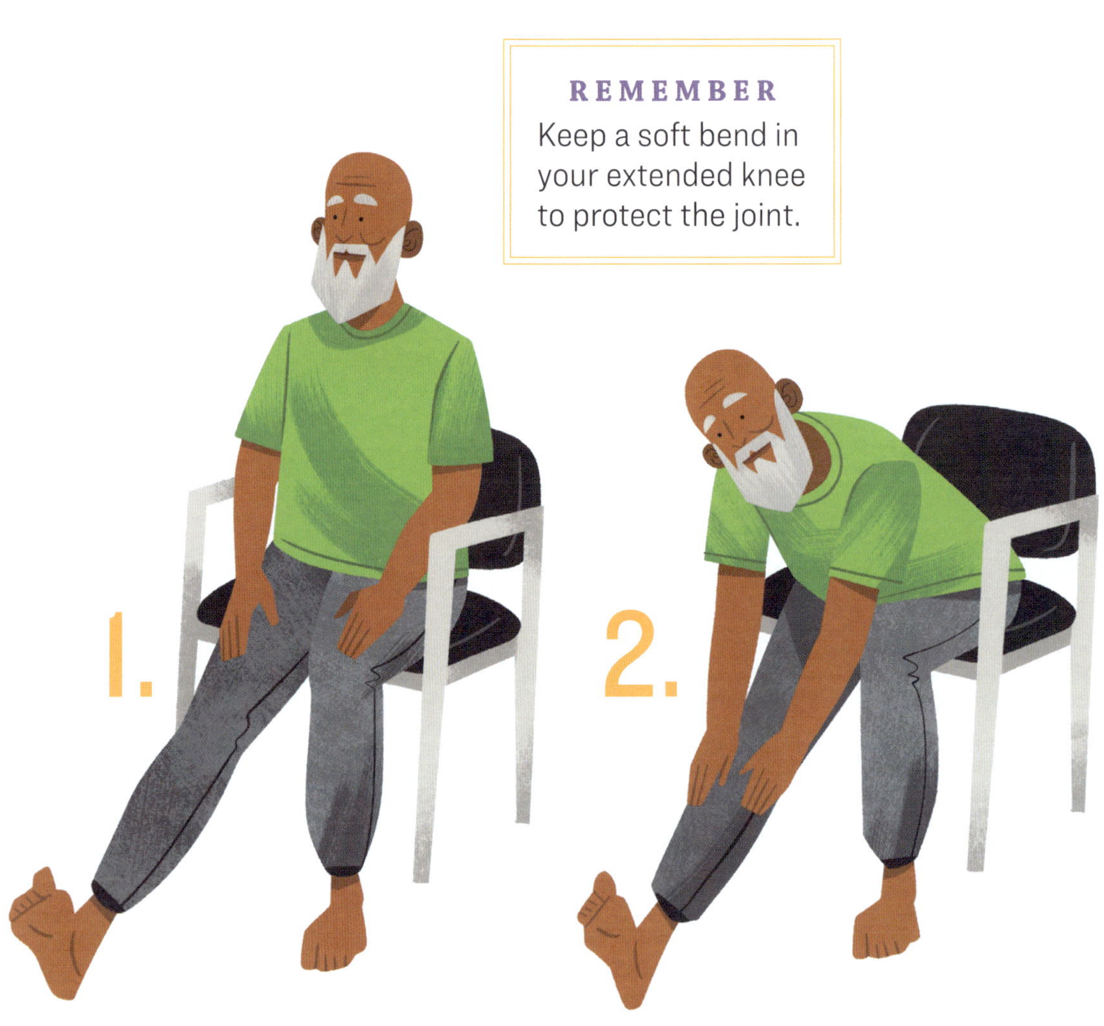

# SEATED FORWARD FOLD WITH LEG EXTENSION

## JANU SIRSASANA

**TARGETED AREAS:** Calves, hamstrings, lower back

Seated Forward Fold with Leg Extension is a perfect way to relieve tension from standing and moving around, like after preparing a holiday feast or touring a museum. I love including this pose in my cooldowns for older adults because it gently stretches the glutes and hamstrings.

### INSTRUCTIONS

1. From Seated Mountain (page 10), inhale and extend your right leg straight out in front of you with the heel resting on the floor and toes pointing toward the ceiling. Keep your left foot firmly on the floor for stability. Lengthen your spine as you sit tall.
2. Exhale as you bend forward from your hips, reaching your hands toward your extended leg and toes.
3. Hold for 3 to 5 rounds of breath. To return, come up on an inhale, keeping a straight spine. Repeat the pose on the other side.

To simplify, instead of reaching forward, place your hands on your hips for stability, or on the thigh of your extended leg. Focus on maintaining a long spine and gently lean forward slightly from your hips.

For a challenge, with your leg extended, lift your heel slightly off the floor. This will activate your legs and core.

**Keep in Mind:** Keep your back straight as you bend at the hips. If you feel discomfort in your lower back, decrease the bend or sit upright.

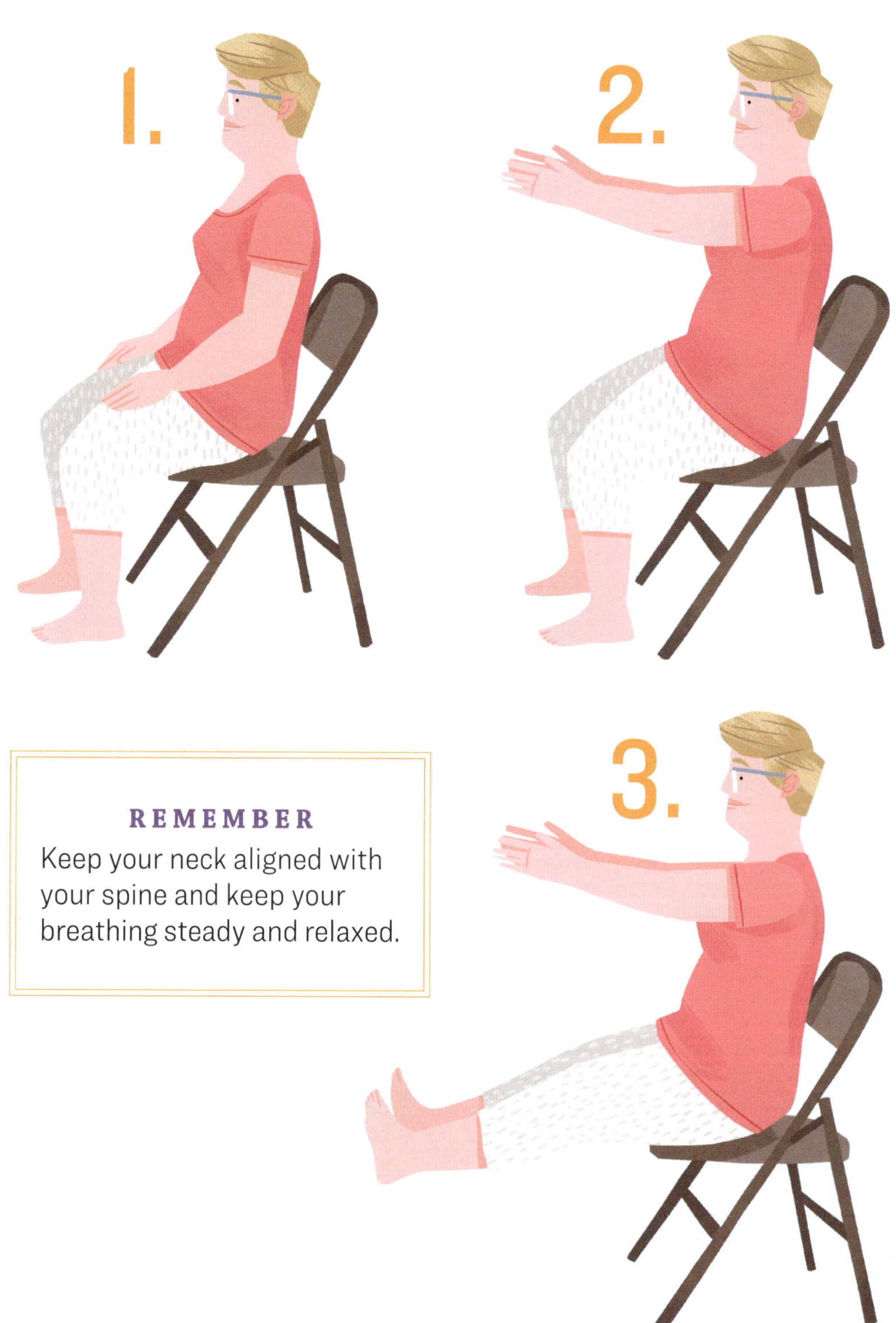


**REMEMBER**

Keep your neck aligned with your spine and keep your breathing steady and relaxed.

# SEATED BOAT

## NAVASANA

**TARGETED AREAS:** Back, core, hips

Seated Boat will help you stay steady as you navigate the seas of daily life. In this pose, your sit bones serve as a fulcrum between your lifted legs and upper body. Your core, hip flexors, and spinal stabilizers activate, contributing to improved balance, posture, and overall mobility. This is one of the more challenging poses in the book, so you might want to experiment with the easier modification. Whichever version works best for you will still provide Seated Boat's full benefits.

### INSTRUCTIONS

1. From Seated Mountain (page 10), sit toward the front of your chair and lean back slightly while maintaining a neutral back.
2. Inhale and extend your arms forward at shoulder height, parallel to the floor, your palms facing each other.
3. Exhale and lift both feet a few inches off the floor, straightening your legs while keeping a soft bend in your knees.
4. Take 3 to 5 rounds of breath, remembering to keep your chest up.

To simplify, lift one foot at a time with a soft bend in the knees and you are leaning back. You can even "march" your feet, lifting one at a time repeatedly.

For a challenge, extend your arms overhead while maintaining a neutral back.

**Keep in Mind:** If you experience discomfort in your back or hips, reduce the range of motion or keep your feet on the floor while leaning back slightly.

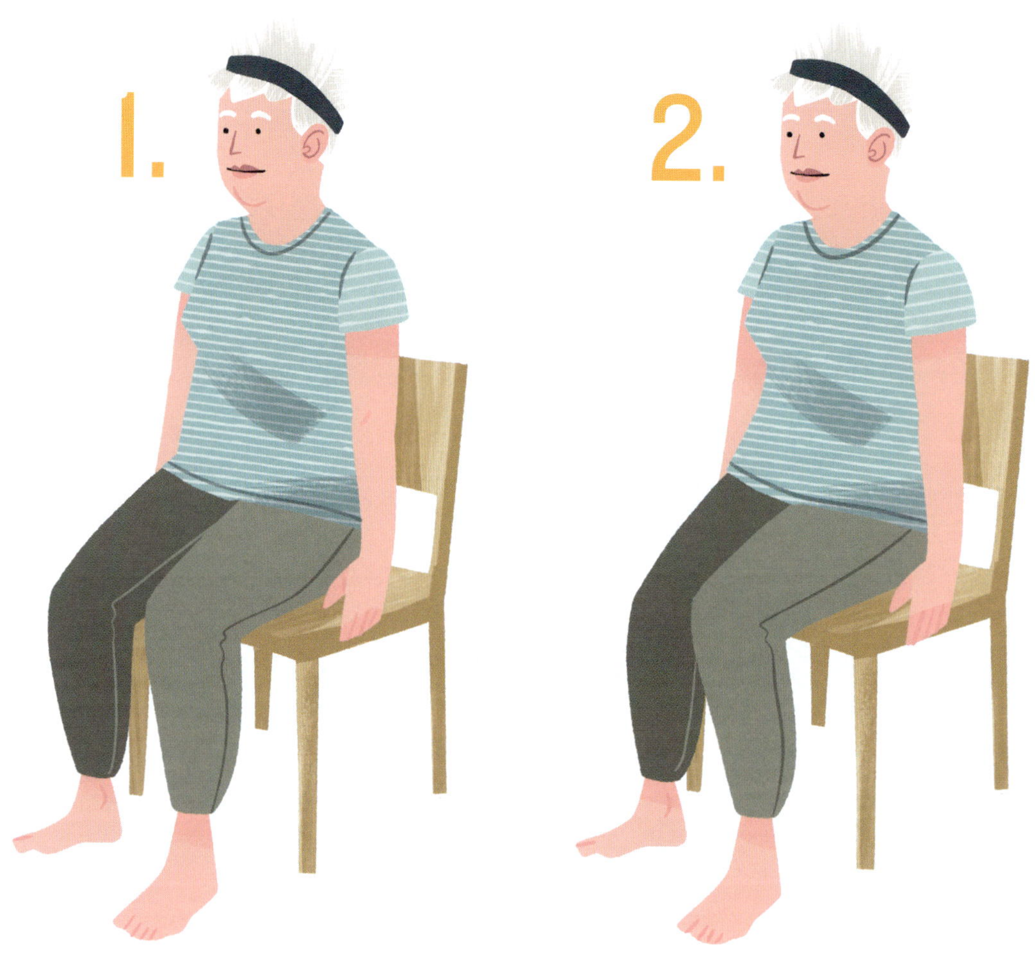


**REMEMBER**

Activate your core, feeling your upper body lift as you squeeze your glutes and thighs.

# SEATED BRIDGE

## SETU BANDHASANA

**TARGETED AREAS:** Core, glutes, hamstrings, hips

Seated Bridge provides a solid foundation by strengthening your lower body, all while you sit in a comfortable chair. In addition to making moving around easier, this gentle move can strengthen pelvic floor function. This pose is similar to Seated Chair (page 56) but it focuses on engaging the glutes.

### INSTRUCTIONS

1. From Seated Mountain (page 10), inhale and place your hands on the sides of the chair, gripping lightly, or keep them on your thighs. You can dig your heels into the floor.
2. Exhale and press firmly through your feet, squeezing your glutes and thighs. Hold this pose for 3 to 5 breaths.

For a challenge, squeeze your glutes and thighs and slightly lift your butt off the chair, activating your arms and shoulders. Keep your neck in line with your spine.

**Keep in Mind:** Squeezing your glutes and thighs is a subtle but powerful move. You should feel your glutes and hamstrings lift and tighten.

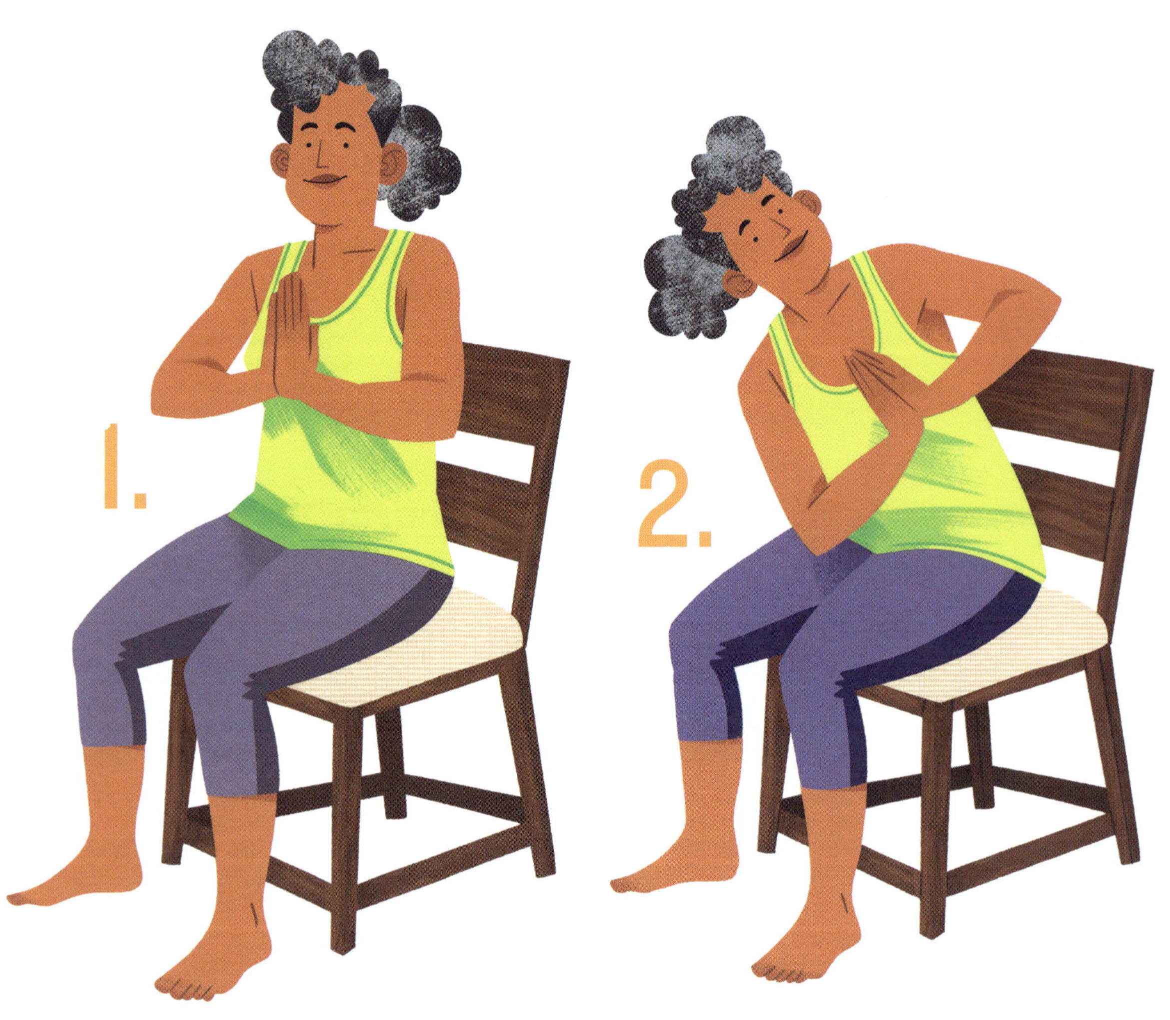


**REMEMBER**

Relax your gaze either forward or over your left shoulder, depending on the comfort of your neck.

# SEATED REVOLVED CHAIR

## PARIVRTTA UTKATASANA

**TARGETED AREAS:** Back, core, shoulders, spine

Let's build on the solid lower-body foundation of Seated Chair (page 56) and add a twist! This pose helps you find a good, supported stretch in your sides and can relieve tension from keeping your arms in the same position for a while, as you might if you're working on the computer or doing sudoku all day.

## INSTRUCTIONS

1. From Seated Mountain (page 10), place your hands in a prayer position at your chest, with your thumbs lightly touching the center of your chest, or sternum.
2. Inhale, lengthening your spine as if a string is pulling the top of your head toward the ceiling. As you exhale, twist your torso to the left, dipping your right elbow down so it's hovering above your left thigh. Keep your left elbow pointing up and behind you, with your palms pressing together.
3. Hold the twist for 3 to 5 rounds of breath, keeping your hips grounded and your knees aligned. With each inhale, lengthen your spine. With each exhale, deepen the twist slightly if you're up for it, being mindful not to force the movement.
4. Repeat on your right side.

To simplify, keep your hands on your thighs while twisting, gazing over your shoulder if possible.

For a challenge, extend your arms outward. With your left arm, reach up, and with your right arm, reach toward the floor, on the outside of your left thigh.

**Keep in Mind:** If you have osteoporosis or spinal issues, check with your healthcare provider before doing this pose. Focus on twisting only as far as your body comfortably allows, without straining your back, neck, or shoulders. If you feel any sharp pain or discomfort, ease out of the twist.

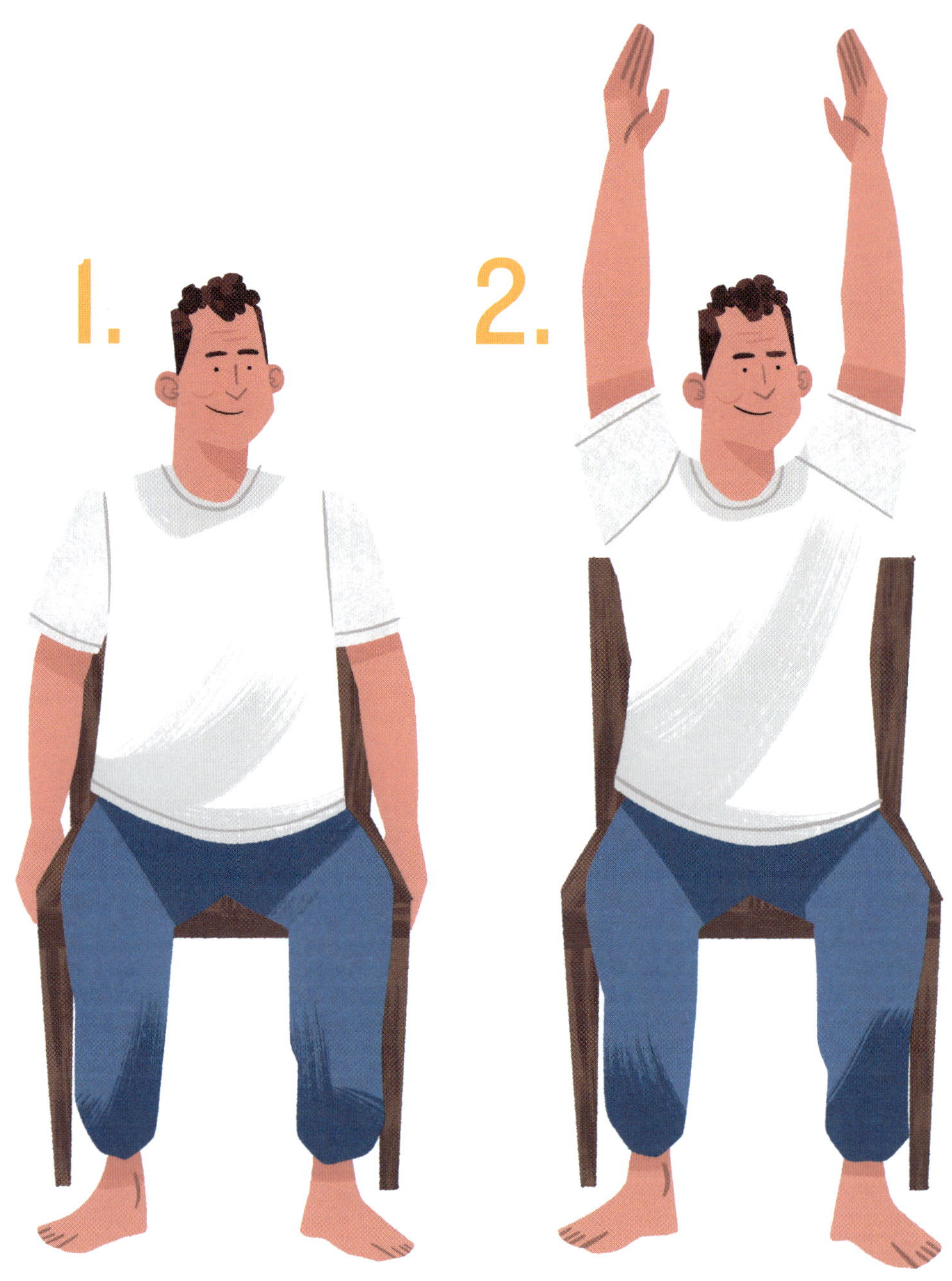


**REMEMBER**

Lengthen your spine with each inhale and keep your core engaged as you exhale.

# SEATED UPWARD SALUTE

## URDHVA HASTASANA

**TARGETED AREAS:** Back, core, neck, shoulders

Lengthening your spine and raising your arms overhead can be an energizing way to greet the day, find some brightness between tasks, and boost lung capacity. Let's salute our mind and body strength.

### INSTRUCTIONS

1. From Seated Mountain (page 10), roll your shoulders back and down to open your chest.
2. Lengthen your spine, imagining a string gently pulling from the top of your head. Inhale and sweep your arms up and overhead, keeping your palms facing each other.
3. Exhale and extend through your fingertips by stretching your fingers wide, reaching toward the ceiling while keeping your shoulders relaxed and away from your ears. Visualize your shoulder blades moving down your back.
4. Hold the position for 3 to 5 rounds of breath. If it's comfortable, gently lift your gaze toward your hands without straining your neck.

To simplify, lift your arms in front of you to shoulder height with soft elbows and palms facing each other for ease.

For a challenge, place your palms together after you raise your arms overhead, to further stretch and strengthen your shoulders and back.

**Keep in Mind:** Keep your movements slow and controlled, focusing on the range of motion in your shoulders. If you feel any discomfort or pain, reduce the height of your arms and focus on maintaining a tall, neutral spine with deep, steady breathing.

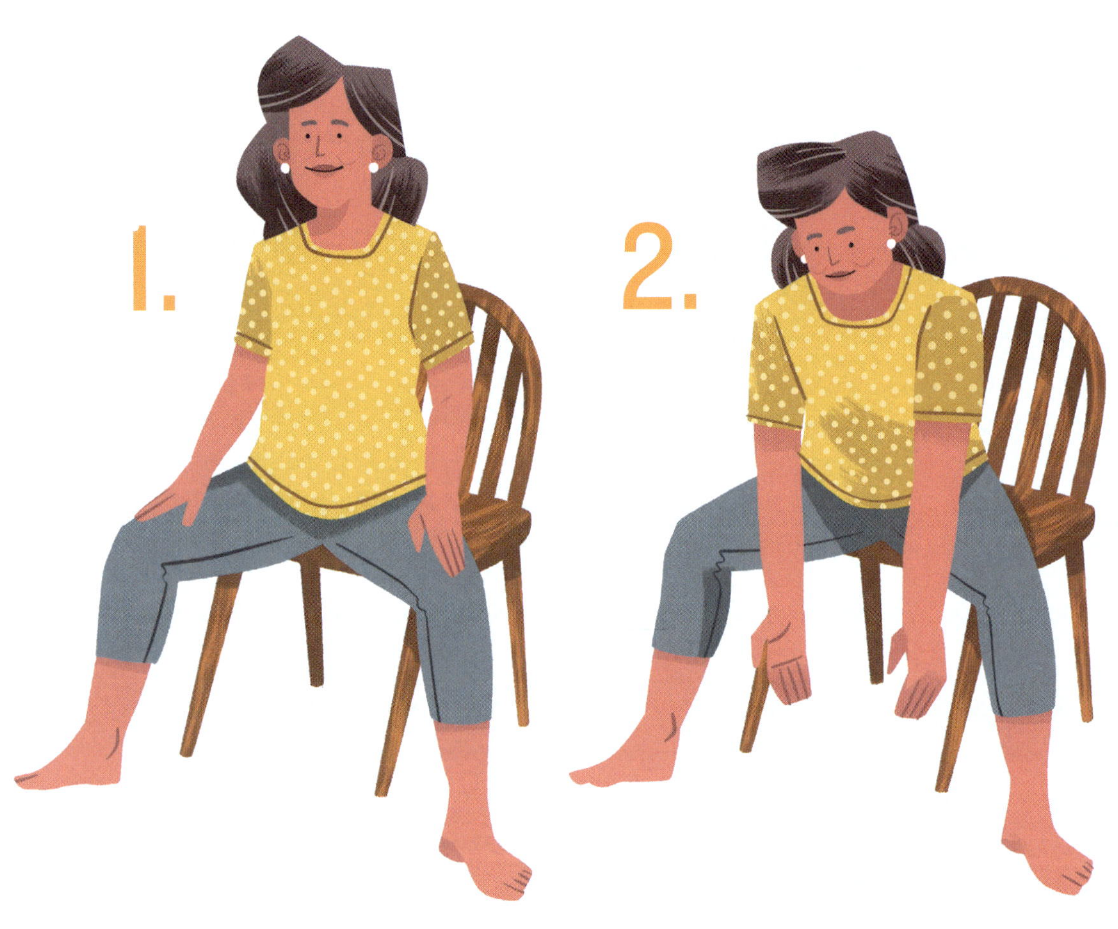


**REMEMBER**

As you bend, pause at a point where you feel a gentle stretch in your inner thighs, hips, and back. Be careful of tipping forward. Start small and experiment with increasing the tilt until you're familiar with the pose.

# SEATED WIDE-ANGLE FORWARD FOLD

## UPAVISTHA KONASANA

**TARGETED AREAS:** Back, hamstrings, hips, inner thighs

Seated Wide-Angle Forward Fold offers the opportunity to stretch your inner thighs and hips and to find length through the spine. As you get more accustomed to the pose, it can make bending at your waist easier, and the stability you build in your lower body and low back can support improved balance and fall-preventing posture.

### INSTRUCTIONS

1. Start in Seated Horse (page 60).
2. Inhale and lengthen your spine, sitting as tall as possible. On an exhale, let a bend start from your hips. Engage your hips and keep your knees moving apart to begin the bend. Keep your back straight as you lower your chest and reach your hands toward the floor. You can rest your hands on a stool or nearby low surface for more support.
3. Stay here for 3 to 5 rounds of breath. On each inhale, focus on lengthening your spine. On each exhale, see if you can relax deeper into the pose. To exit the pose, strongly engage your core and come up on an inhale with a straight spine. Imagine someone is pushing you up by the front of your shoulders.

For a challenge, to strengthen your calves, bend your knees sixty to ninety degrees with your feet flat on the floor and lift your heels as you fold.

**Keep in Mind:** If you feel discomfort in your hamstrings, inner thighs, or back, move your legs closer together. As with all folding poses, keep your head above or in line with your heart as you fold if you have heart or other health issues.

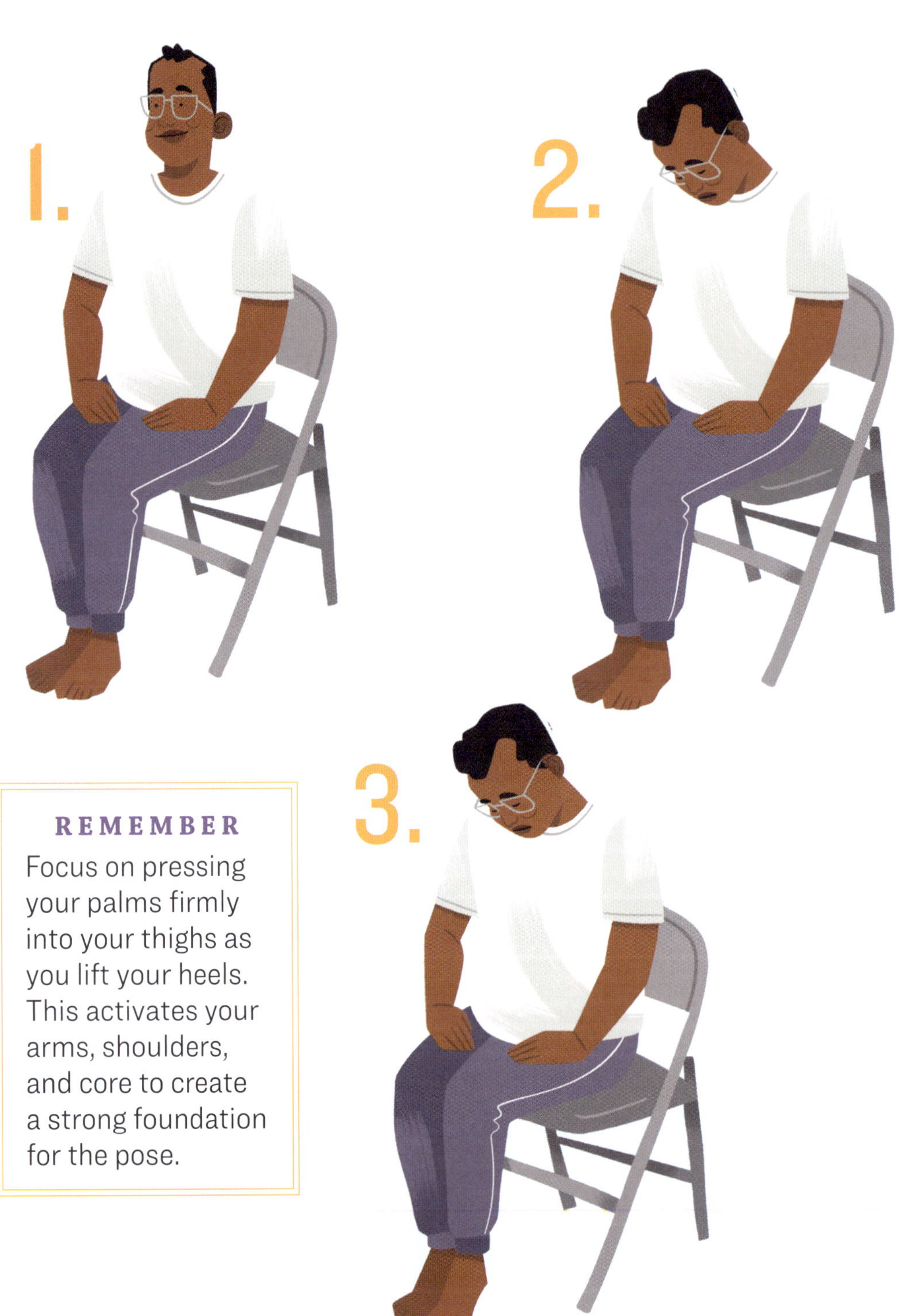


**REMEMBER**

Focus on pressing your palms firmly into your thighs as you lift your heels. This activates your arms, shoulders, and core to create a strong foundation for the pose.

# SEATED CROW

## BAKASANA

**TARGETED AREAS:** Arms, back, calves, core, feet, legs, shoulders

This pose echoes a shape from Seated Cat-Cow (page 14): a rounded shape that engages the whole body. Even your ankles get in on the action when you lift your heels—helping increase the range of motion in the ankles and strengthening calves and lower legs—giving you surer footing. Some benefits to crow about!

### INSTRUCTIONS

1. Inhale and bring your feet together with the inside of your knees, heels, and base of your big toes touching. Place your hands on your thighs, fingers pointing inward. Keep a soft bend in your elbows and point them outward.
2. Exhale, dropping your chin toward your chest to elongate the back of your neck and round your back, pulling your belly button into your spine. Imagine drawing your shoulders to your hips to create a compact shape.
3. Lift your heels off the ground, coming onto the balls of your feet. Press your hands to your thighs for stability.
4. Maintain this pose for 3 to 5 rounds of breath while pressing your hands into your thighs.

To simplify, keep your heels hip-width apart and lift one foot at a time, squeezing your knees toward each other.

For a challenge, lift both feet slightly off the floor, balancing on your sit bones/glutes.

**Keep in Mind:** Sit toward the center of the chair seat, not too close to the edge, to ensure better stability and reduce the risk of tipping forward during the pose. Keep shoulders relaxed away from your cars as you push down on your thighs.

1.

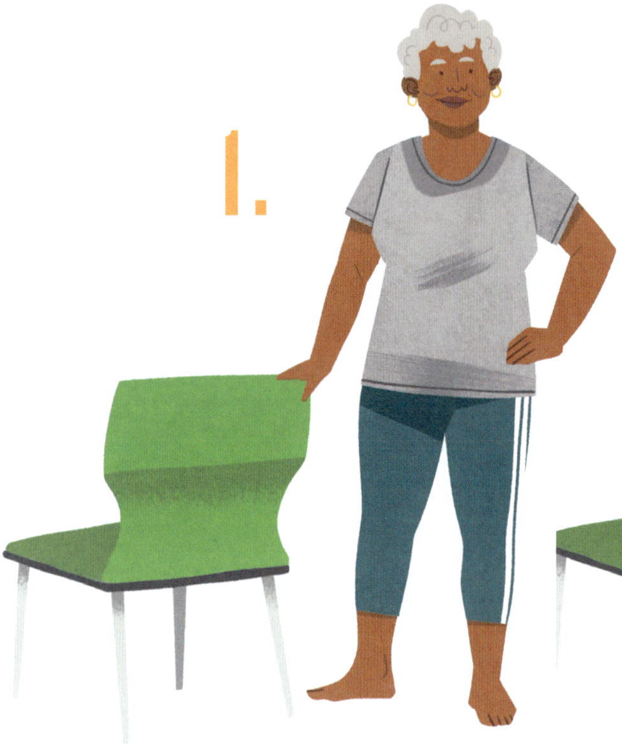

2.

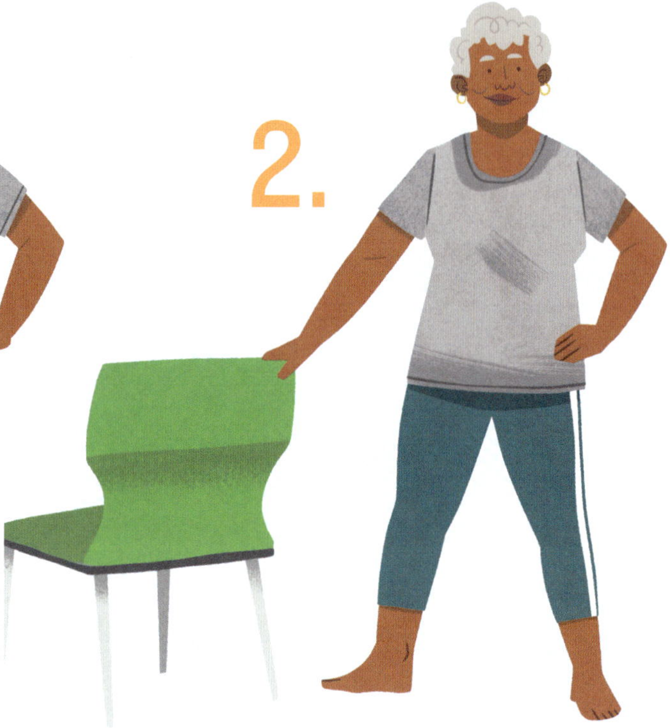

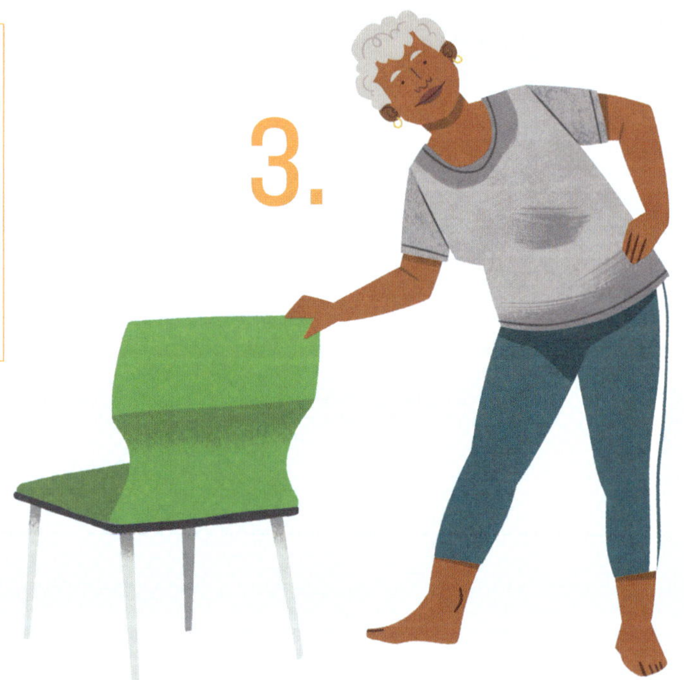


**REMEMBER**

Keep a soft bend in your knees to protect your joints and engage your quadriceps so your kneecaps lift.

# STANDING TRIANGLE

## TRIKONASANA

**TARGETED AREAS:** Arms, core, legs, shoulders

I love doing this sideways pose during the day, after sitting at the computer for hours, and before I sleep at night. It relieves neck and shoulder tightness and can help reduce back pain by opening up the lower body, especially the hips.

## INSTRUCTIONS

1. Stand sideways at the back of your chair with your right hand resting on top of it. The toes of your right foot should point toward the chair. Place your left hand on your hip.
2. Inhale and step your left foot out to the side, wider than your left hip, aligning your left arch with your right heel. Turn the left foot toward the chair at a 45-degree angle, as comfortable, or let toes point straight out. Your right arm should have a soft bend in the elbow.
3. Exhale and shift your left hip to the left, feeling the stretch in your left side: legs, hip, and torso. Gaze forward or upward while keeping your neck in alignment with your spine. You can look down if you feel too much tension in your neck.
4. Hold the pose for 3 to 5 rounds of breath and switch sides.

To simplify, sit with your feet wider than shoulder-width apart, knees over ankles, hands on hips. Lean right, straightening your right arm and reaching toward the floor or low support like a stool, ottoman, or yoga block.

For a challenge, extend the left arm up from the position on your hip, deepening the stretch.

**Keep in Mind:** This pose is a lateral or sideways move—there should be no bending or twisting of the spine. Keep your back straight, gently bending to the side at the hip.

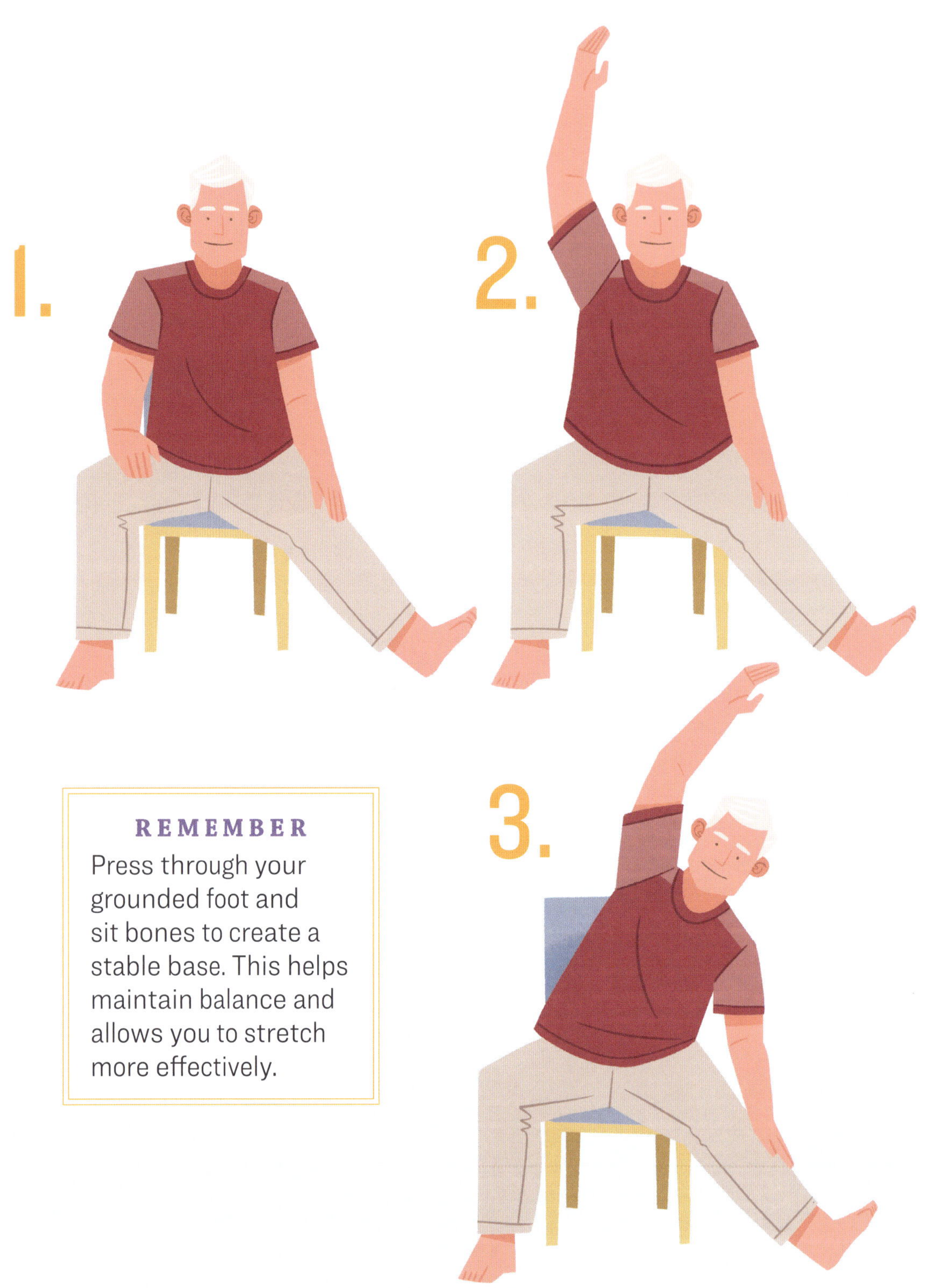


**REMEMBER**

Press through your grounded foot and sit bones to create a stable base. This helps maintain balance and allows you to stretch more effectively.

# SEATED GATE

## PARIGHASANA

**TARGETED AREAS:** Back, core, hips, legs

Open the gate and welcome in easier bends, steadiness, and improved energy. This pose enhances hip and side-body flexibility and reduces stiffness, enabling you to stay active throughout your day.

### INSTRUCTIONS

1. From Seated Mountain (page 10), sit slightly forward on the seat. Extend your left leg out to the side with a soft bend in the knee, heel on the floor and toes pointing up. Keep your right foot flat on the floor for stability.
2. Place your left hand lightly on your left thigh for support. Inhale as you raise your right arm overhead, reaching toward the ceiling with your palm facing inward. Your neck should be in line with the spine, looking forward. If you feel tension in your neck, you may look down.
3. Exhale as you tilt your torso left, keeping your back straight, toward your extended left leg. You should feel a stretch along the right side of your body. Do not put any pressure on the knee of your extended leg.
4. Hold the pose for 3 to 5 rounds of breath, coming up slowly on an inhale. Switch sides.

To simplify, bend your left knee with your foot flat on the floor, knee over ankle. Place your left hand on your left thigh and right hand on your hip. Lean to your left.

For a challenge, lift your extended leg slightly off the floor to engage your leg and core.

**Keep in Mind:** The bending motion originates at your hips, not your shoulders. Avoid slouching forward by lifting your chest toward the ceiling as you bend to the side.

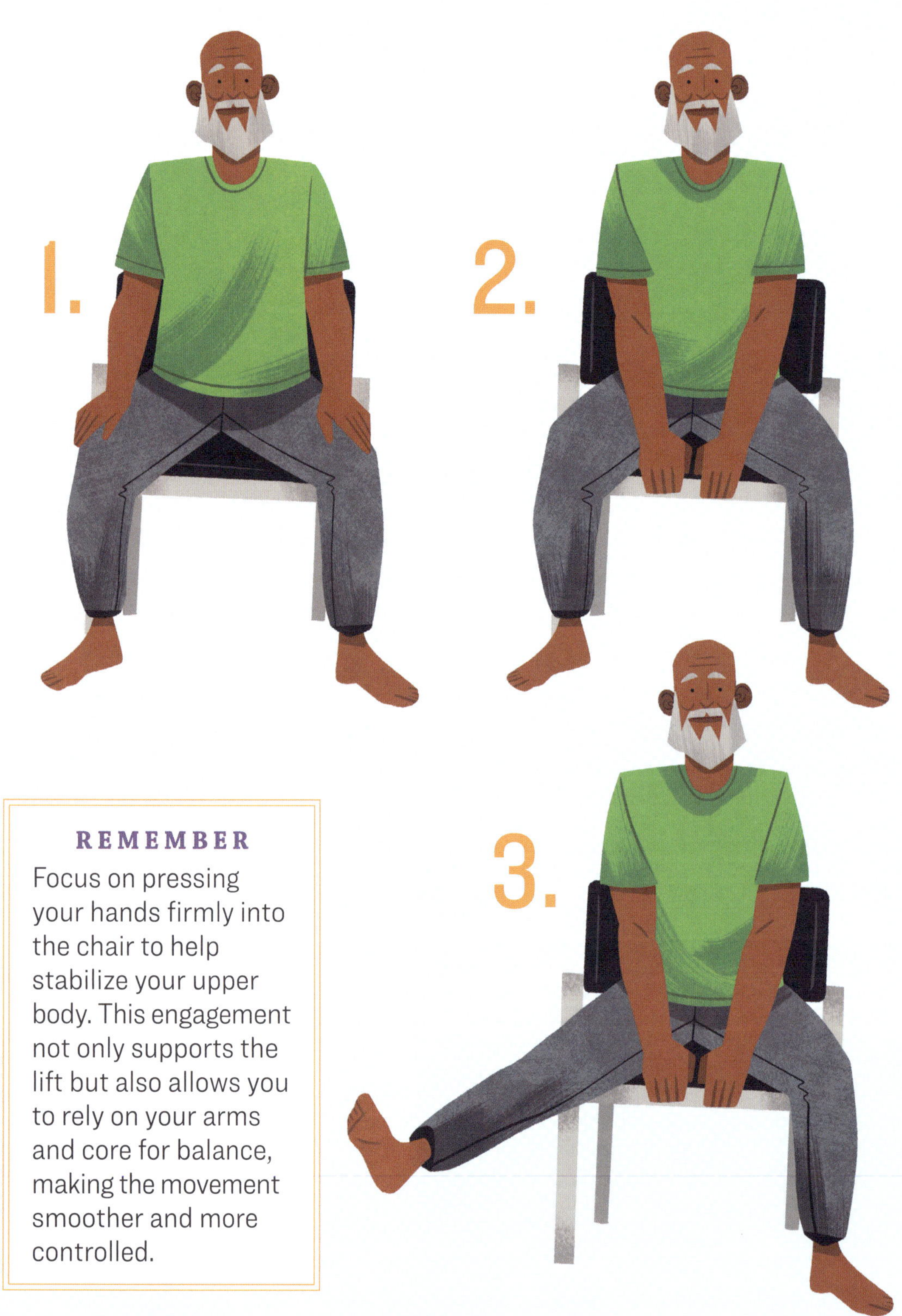


**REMEMBER**

Focus on pressing your hands firmly into the chair to help stabilize your upper body. This engagement not only supports the lift but also allows you to rely on your arms and core for balance, making the movement smoother and more controlled.

# SEATED FIREFLY

## TITTIBHASANA

**TARGETED AREAS:** Core, hip flexors, hips, legs, thighs, upper back

Find lightness and glide through daily tasks with Seated Firefly! Whether you want to work toward moving more smoothly when bending down and straightening to pick up a pet, stepping over a stream on a hike, tending to your garden, or reorganizing the closet, this pose can help you get there.

### INSTRUCTIONS

1. Start in Seated Horse (page 60), sitting farther back in your chair. Let your legs rest wider than hip-width apart, knees bent, with your feet flat on the floor. Point your toes outward to create a stable base and ensure comfort in your hips.
2. Inhale and place your hands on the chair between your legs. Keep your back straight, with slightly bent elbows, even if you have to lean slightly forward.
3. Exhale and straighten your right leg with a soft bend in the knee, then lift it off the floor with your toes pointing up to ceiling. Hold this position while sitting tall and engaging your core and arms. Remember to breathe.
4. Take 3 to 5 rounds of breath, focusing on staying upright with your core engaged, trying not to lean over to one side. Switch sides.

To simplify, keep the right leg straight but engage the muscles *as if* you are going to lift that leg up off the floor.

For a challenge, lift both feet off the floor, toes pointed, to engage the entire leg, or point your toes up to stretch the back of your legs.

**Keep in Mind:** Keep your back straight! Don't round your shoulders or lean too far forward. This ensures proper alignment and minimizes strain on your lower back, reducing the risk of discomfort or injury.

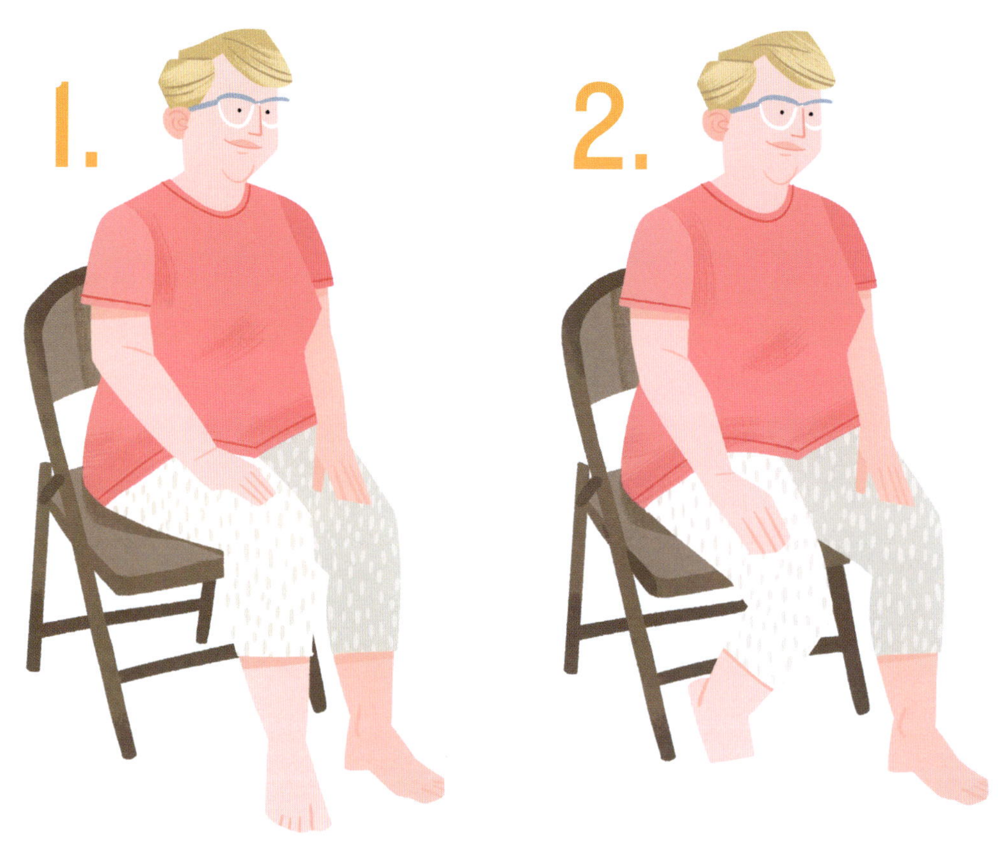


**REMEMBER**

To protect your joints, keep your toes in line with your ankles and knees, with no inward or outward rotation.

# SEATED HERO

## VIRASANA

**TARGETED AREAS:** Ankles, feet, front thighs, shins

Seated Hero is perfect for improving joint stability and for tending to your feet. It stretches the tops and arches of your feet and builds ankle flexibility. Even if you're simply sitting at the kitchen table talking after a meal, you can take a moment to be a Hero.

### INSTRUCTIONS

1. From Seated Mountain (page 10), inhale and position yourself slightly forward on the chair to allow room for your hips to open comfortably. Rest your hands on your thighs with palms down.
2. Place the top of your foot on the floor by tucking your toes under the chair, exhale, and slide one foot slightly back, behind the knee of the same leg. Press the top of your foot down gently to stretch it. Sit tall, engage your core, and keep your spine elongated and shoulders relaxed. Hold the sides of the chair for support, if needed, or rest your hands on your thighs.
3. Take 3 to 5 rounds of breath to settle into the stretch, which you should feel in the top of the foot, ankle, and shin. Repeat with the other foot.

To simplify, sit with your feet hip-width apart and curl your toes under, with your heels lightly resting on the floor.

For a challenge, slide your feet farther back and raise your arms overhead to engage your core and upper body.

**Keep in Mind:** If you have limited flexibility in your feet, don't force the stretch. Listen to your body and make adjustments for comfort.

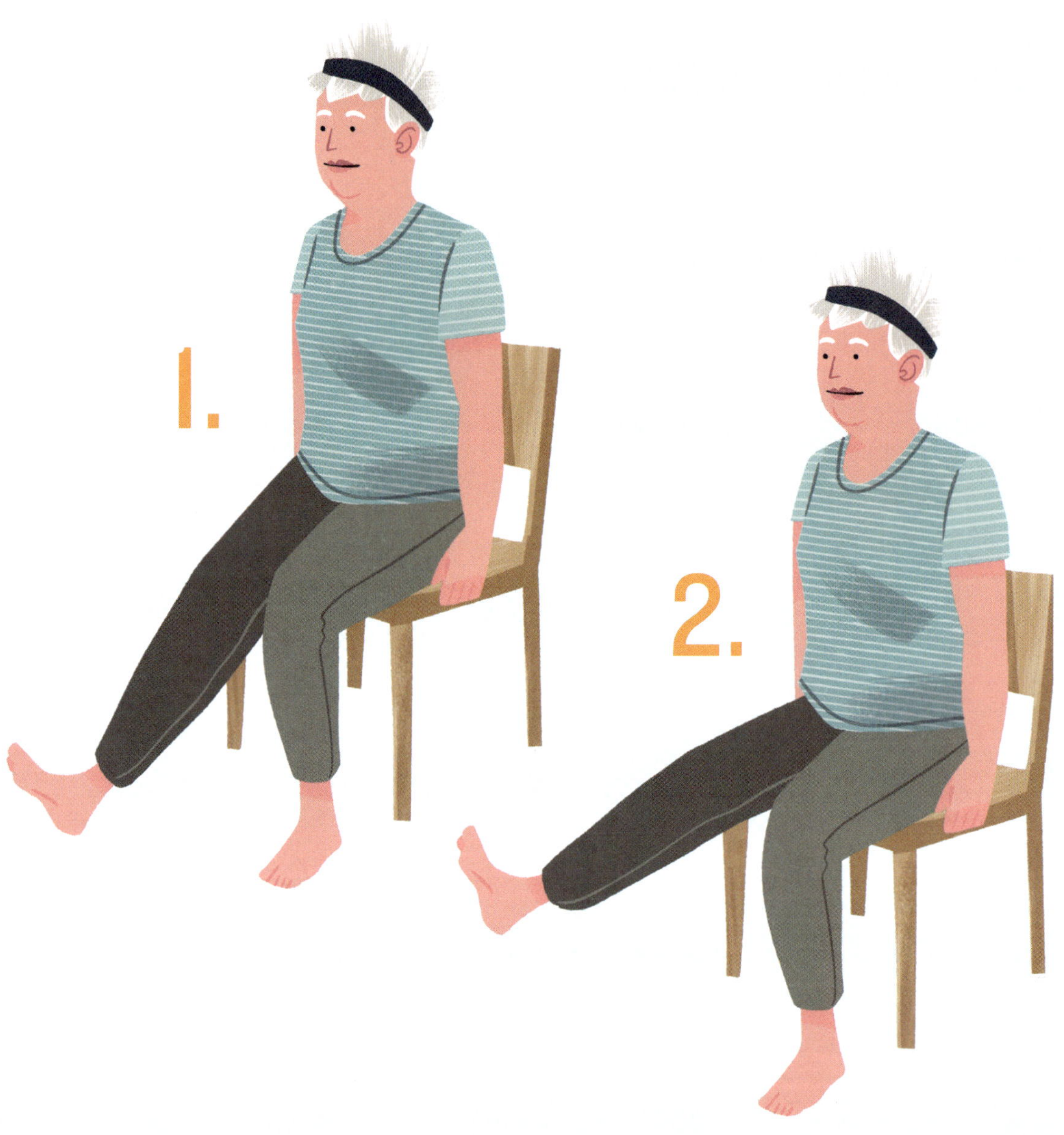


**REMEMBER**

The lifting motion of your extended leg originates in your hip and quadriceps, not your knee.

# SEATED LEG LIFT

## UTTANPADASANA

**TARGETED AREAS:** Ankles, calves, core, front thighs, hips

This is a great "anytime, anywhere" pose that can give your legs a boost while you drink your morning coffee or watch your favorite show! Strengthen your legs, hips, and core while being gentle on your knees and joints.

### INSTRUCTIONS

1. Start in Seated Calf and Toe Stretch (page 24).
2. Exhale and lift your right leg with a soft bend in the knee until your right thigh is level with your left thigh or to a comfortable level. Even lifting your leg a couple of inches off the floor can be challenging! Take 3 to 5 rounds of breath.
3. Lower your heel back to the floor with control.
4. Repeat 3 to 5 times and switch to the other leg.

To simplify, keep your feet flat on the floor and flex one ankle at a time or both together. Alternatively, engage the straight leg *as if* lifting it. Imagine being able to slide a piece of paper under your heel.

For a challenge, hold a towel or belt in both hands and place it under the ball of the lifted foot to deepen the stretch.

**Keep in Mind:** To stay stable, ensure your back stays straight and don't lean back. Keep a soft bend in your knee throughout the pose to make sure it doesn't lock. If extra support is needed, place your hands on the sides of the chair.

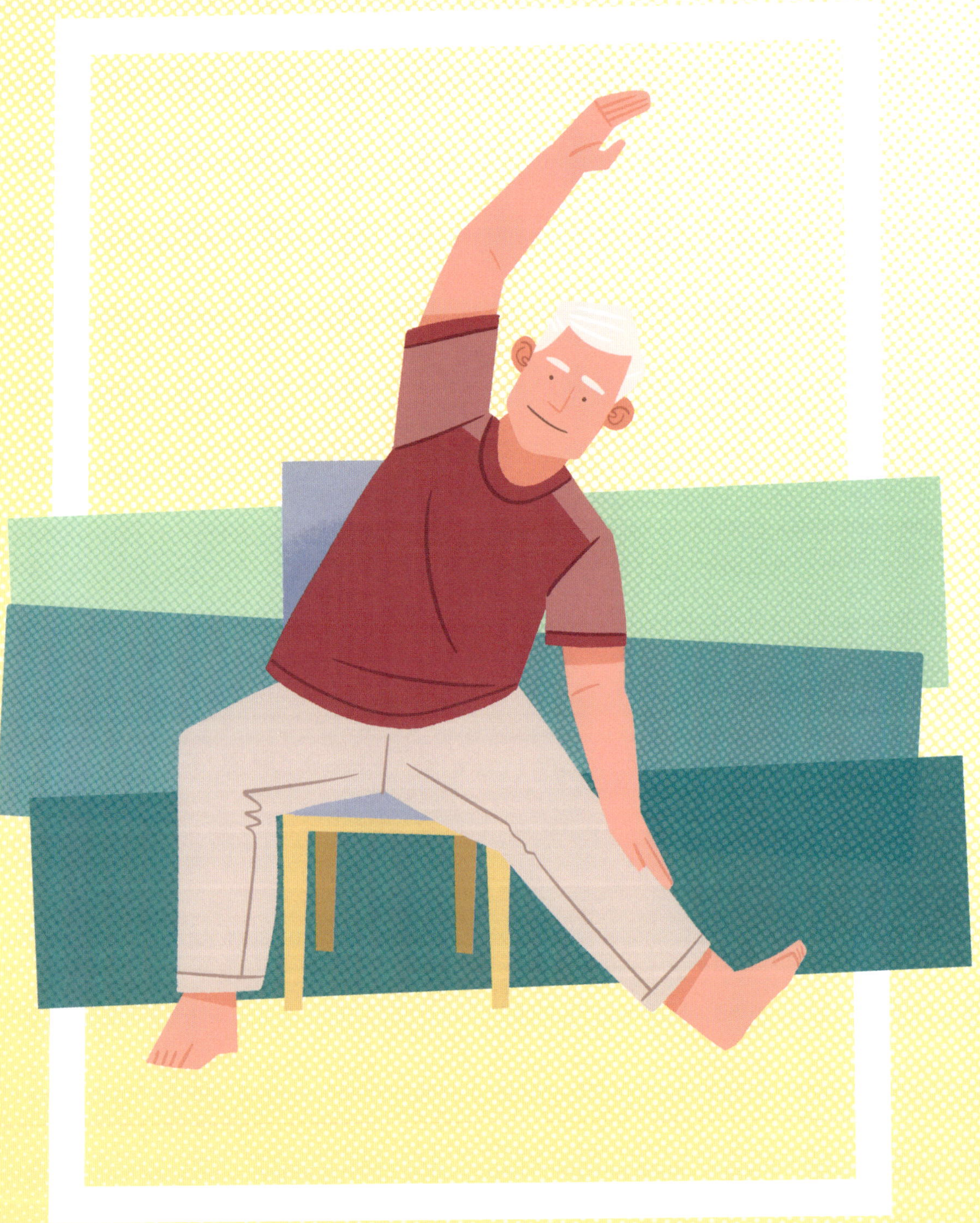

PART THREE

# CHAIR YOGA SEQUENCES

**IF YOU'RE READY** to add a little more structure to your practice, this section goes over twenty-five fun, easy-to-follow sequences. Each sequence features two to four poses from part 2 and targets key areas like your hips, legs, or overall strength and energy. These sequences are designed to flow smoothly from one pose to the next. Some poses naturally transition to other poses, while others move to the foundational Seated Mountain Pose (page 10) before moving on to the next pose. Each sequence is designed to be done twice to achieve a ten-minute session.

Have fun with your practice! You can choose to do just one sequence or even combine a few sequences if you're feeling adventurous. Remember to take it at your own pace—there's no need to rush. Move gently, transition smoothly, and listen to your body. If something doesn't feel quite right, make adjustments for your comfort. This is your time to move, breathe, and feel fantastic on your own terms!

## WARM UP: GENTLY WAKE UP

1\. **Seated Cat-Cow**
PAGE 14

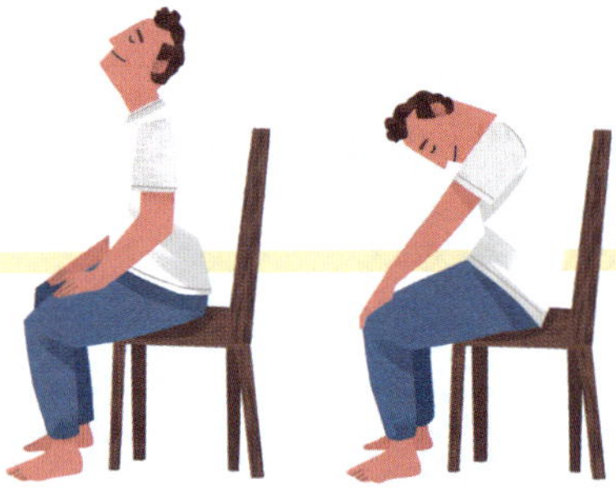

2\. **Seated Calf and Toe Stretch**
PAGE 24

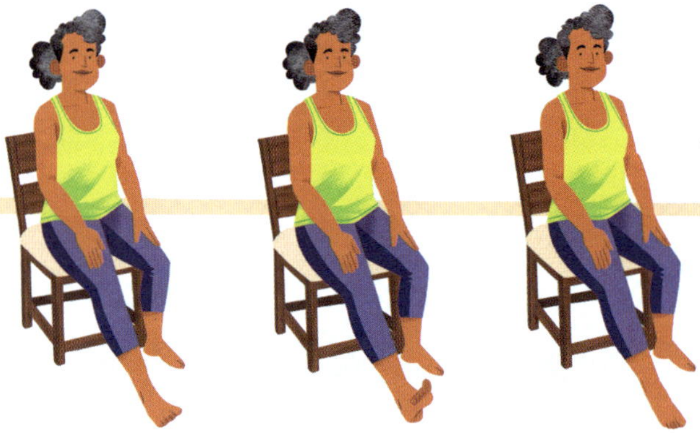

## COOL DOWN: RELAX AND RESTORE

1\. **Seated Forward Fold**
PAGE 28

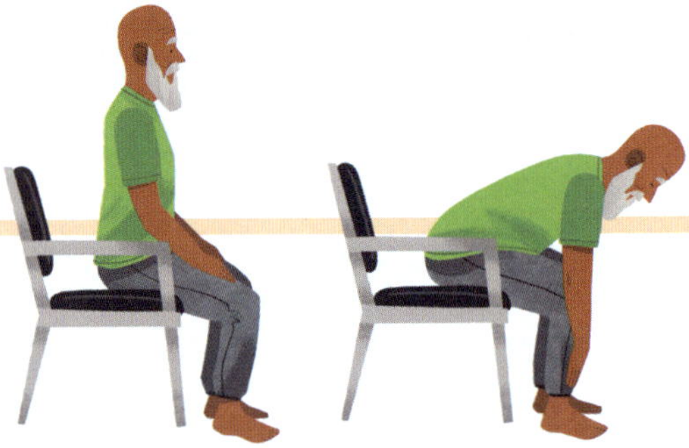

2\. **Seated Rest**
PAGE 16

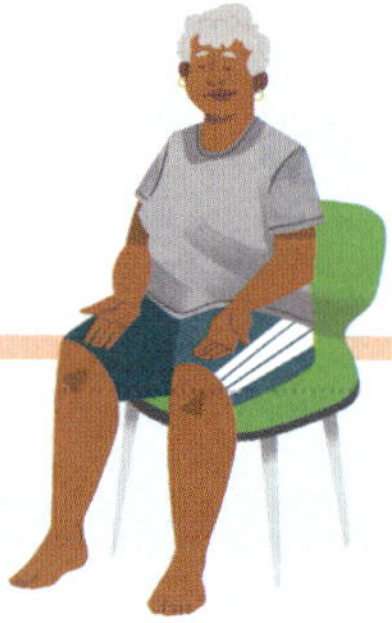

# WARM UP AND COOL DOWN

**TARGETED BENEFITS:** Mobility and Movement

Warming up your muscles and joints before a session and dialing it down after you're done helps prevent injury while calming your mind and body. Warm up and cool down to bookend your practice or on do either part of this sequence on its own to bring energy or relaxation into your day.

## WARM-UP SEQUENCE

1. **SEATED CAT-COW:** Repeat 5 times.
2. **SEATED CALF AND TOE STRETCH:** Repeat 5 times with each foot.

## COOLDOWN SEQUENCE

1. **SEATED FORWARD FOLD:** Do 3 to 5 rounds of breath.
2. **SEATED SAVASANA:** Breathe deeply for 1 to 3 minutes.

**Remember:** Focus on breathing during these poses to deepen your stretches and relaxation.

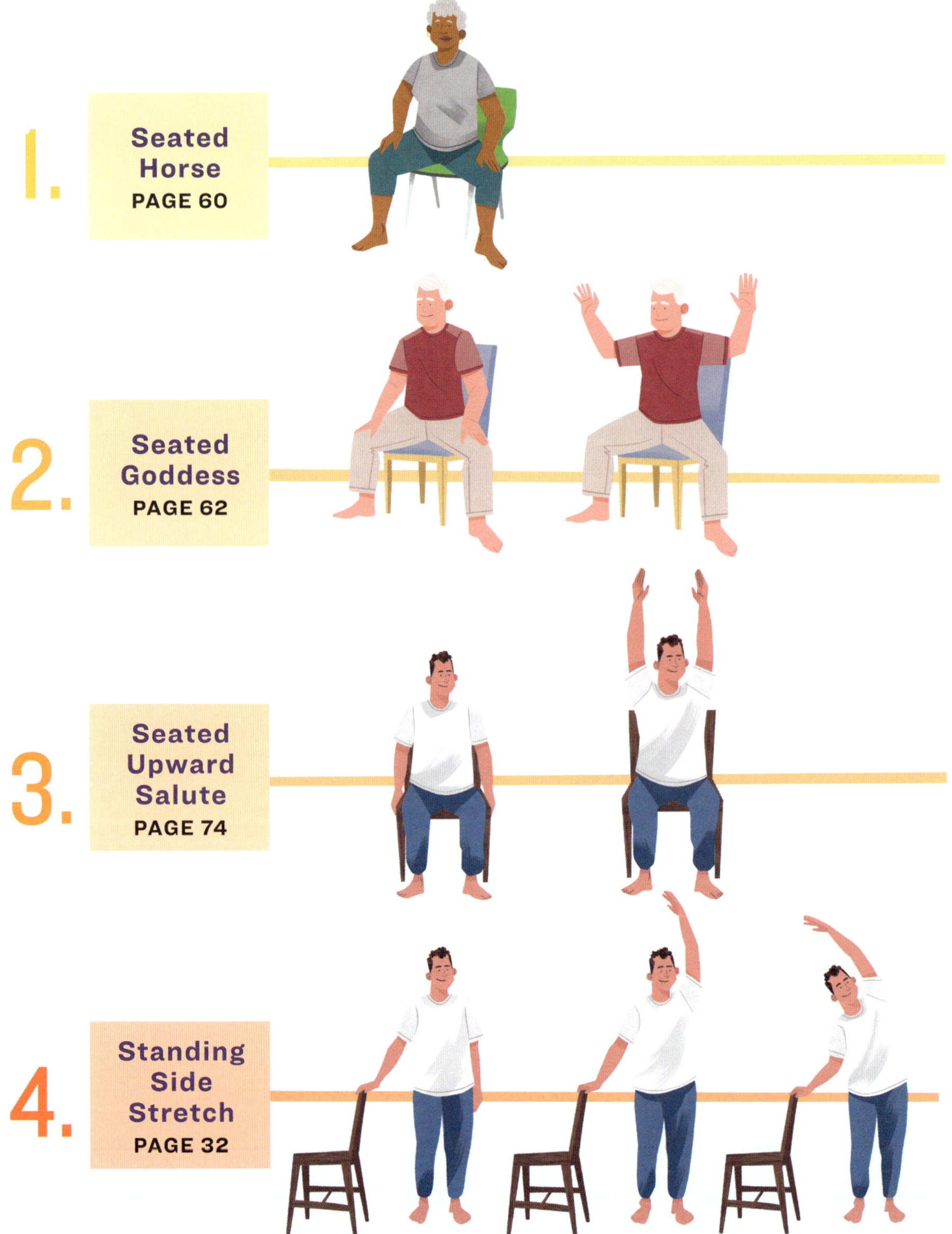
1.
Seated Horse
PAGE 60
2.
Seated Goddess
PAGE 62
3.
Seated Upward Salute
PAGE 74
4.
Standing Side Stretch
PAGE 32

# ENERGIZING BOOST

**TARGETED BENEFITS:** Mobility and Movement

This sequence helps you build strength, balance, and confidence for daily tasks like standing up, walking, and reaching. It strengthens your legs, core, and shoulders while improving posture and focus. Try it in the morning to wake up your body or during the day for an energy boost. Practice it every day or at least three to four times a week.

## THE SEQUENCE

1. **SEATED HORSE:** Hold for 3 to 5 rounds of breath and switch sides.
2. **SEATED GODDESS:** Hold for 3 to 5 rounds of breath.
3. **SEATED UPWARD SALUTE:** Hold for 3 to 5 rounds of breath.
4. **STANDING SIDE STRETCH:** Hold for 3 to 5 rounds of breath and switch sides.

**Remember:** To transition from seated to standing, exhale from Seated Upward Salute, inhale, place your hands on your thighs, and bend at your hips, keeping your back straight. Exhale and press your feet into the floor to stand and set up Standing Side Stretch.

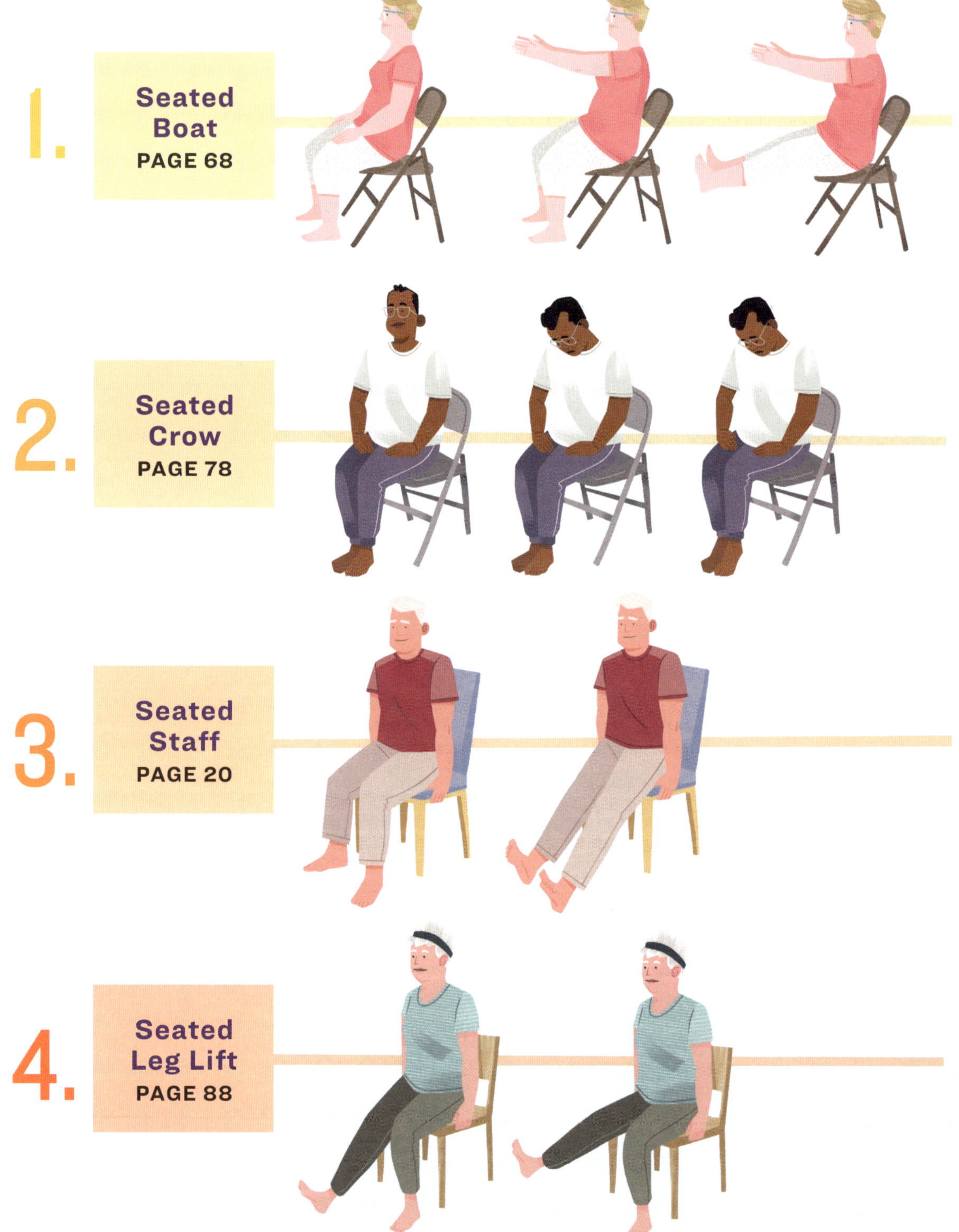
1.
Seated Boat
PAGE 68
2.
Seated Crow
PAGE 78
3.
Seated Staff
PAGE 20
4.
Seated Leg Lift
PAGE 88

# CORE ACTIVATOR

**TARGETED BENEFITS:** Balance and Fall Prevention, Muscle Endurance and Strength

Do you want to move with ease with everything you do? Activate your core and stand tall. A strong core is essential for stability, posture, and movement, and this sequence helps you build that strength. Each pose is designed to engage the muscles in your abdomen, back, and sides, supporting your spine and protecting your lower back from strain. You'll find that tasks like bending, standing, or even reaching for something overhead become easier and safer. Do this sequence any time of day or add to your workout routine to boost your core.

## THE SEQUENCE

1. **SEATED BOAT:** Do 3 rounds of breath.
2. **SEATED CROW:** Do 3 rounds of breath.
3. **SEATED STAFF:** Do 5 rounds of breath.
4. **SEATED LEG LIFT:** Do 5 rounds of breath and switch legs.

**Remember:** Stay aligned by imagining your head over your heart, your heart over your pelvis, and the crown of your head reaching toward the sky. You should feel your abdominal muscles activate.

1. **Seated Pigeon**
**PAGE 50**

2. **Seated Butterfly**
**PAGE 22**

3. **Seated Low Lunge**
**PAGE 18**

4. **Seated Firefly**
**PAGE 84**

# HIP OPENER FLOW

**TARGETED BENEFITS:** Joint Health, Mobility and Movement, Relief of Aches and Pains

Sitting too much can lead to hip tightness, which can cause lower back tension and affect your range of motion. Looser, more flexible hips can reduce stiffness and discomfort, improve posture, and help you walk, bend, and sit more easily. This sequence improves hip mobility, loosens tight muscles, and enhances flexibility, making it easier to move comfortably. It's also excellent for improving posture and reducing pressure on your knees and back. Whether you've been sitting too long or need a gentle stretch after a walk, this flow will leave you feeling refreshed. Practice three to four times a week.

## THE SEQUENCE

1. **SEATED PIGEON:** Hold for 3 rounds of breath and switch legs.
2. **SEATED BUTTERFLY:** Maintain active or holding pose for 20 seconds.
3. **SEATED LOW LUNGE:** Repeat 3 times and switch legs.
4. **SEATED FIREFLY:** Hold for 3 rounds of breath.

**Remember:** To engage your core and avoid rounding your back, sit tall throughout this entire sequence.

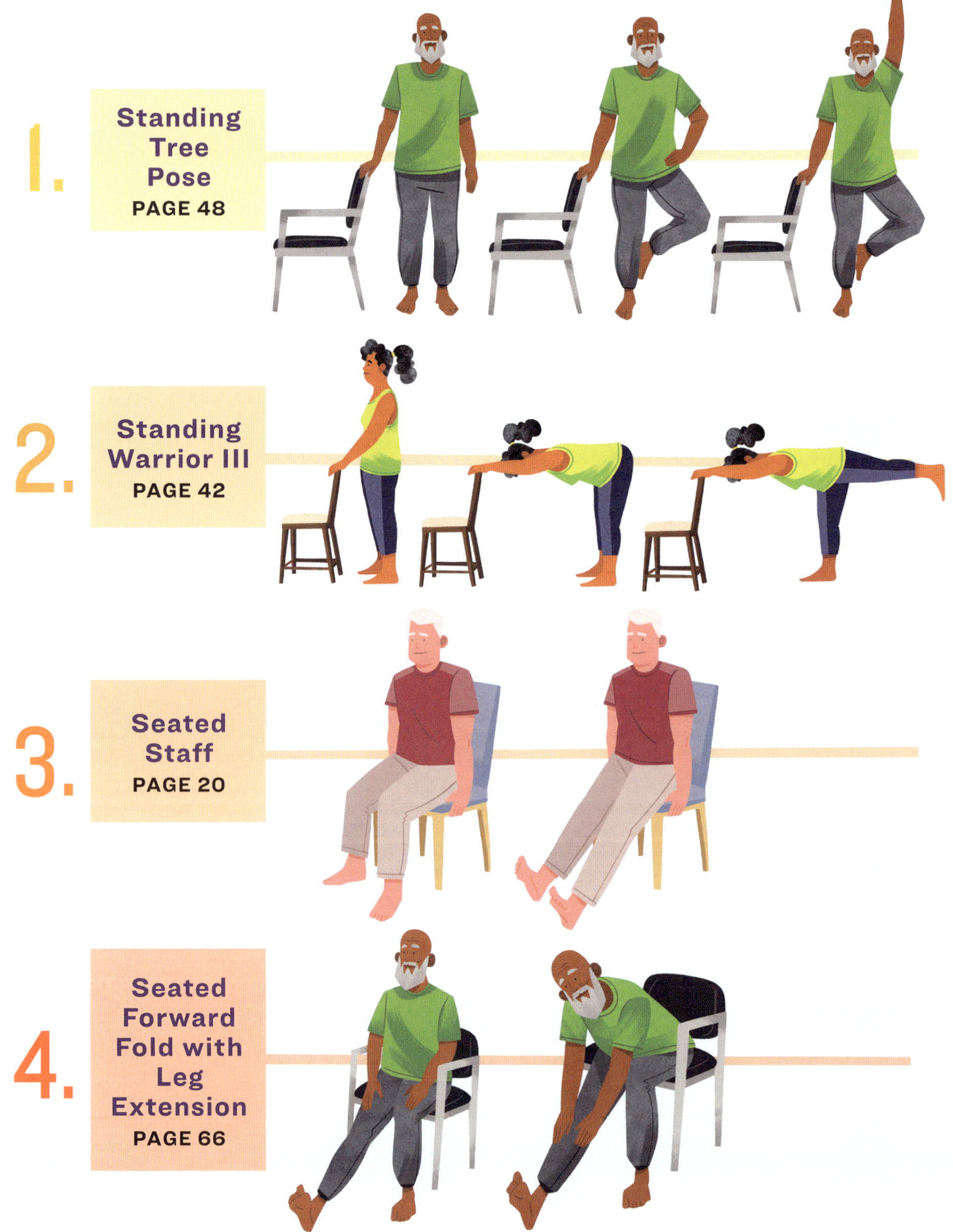
1.
Standing Tree Pose
PAGE 48
2.
Standing Warrior III
PAGE 42
3.
Seated Staff
PAGE 20
4.
Seated Forward Fold with Leg Extension
PAGE 66

# LEG DAY BOOST

**TARGETED BENEFITS:** Mobility and Movement, Muscle Endurance and Strength

Strong legs are the foundation of steady, confident movement, and this sequence is all about strengthening your thighs, calves, and glutes. By focusing on controlled movements, you'll also enhance your balance. The poses in this flow support bone health and build muscle mass, which is vital for maintaining mobility. Over time, you'll feel more confident and capable, whether you're walking, gardening, or simply enjoying time on your feet. Practice three to four times a week, any time of day or after a walk, to boost leg strength.

## THE SEQUENCE

1. **STANDING TREE:** Hold for 3 rounds of breath.
2. **STANDING WARRIOR III:** Hold for 3 rounds of breath.
3. **SEATED STAFF:** Hold for 5 rounds of breath.
4. **SEATED FORWARD FOLD WITH LEG EXTENSION:** Hold for 5 rounds of breath.
5. Repeat the full sequence, switching sides with Standing Tree, Standing Warrior III, and Seated Forward Fold with Leg Extension.

**Remember:** Focus on pressing firmly through your feet during each pose—it helps activate your leg muscles and improves stability. Keep your movements controlled and steady, and don't forget to engage your core for extra support. Remember, strength builds over time, so be patient and consistent.

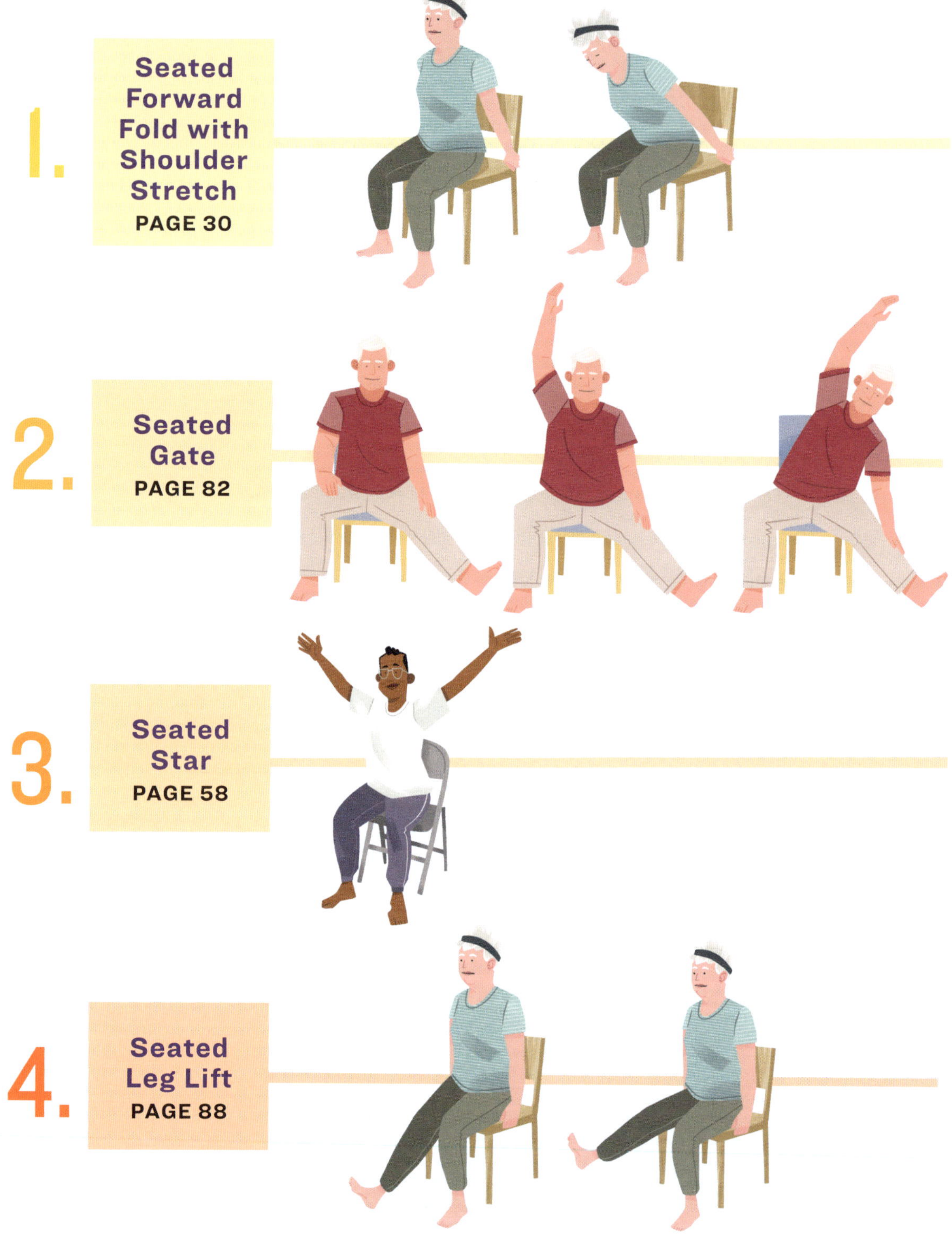

1. **Seated Forward Fold with Shoulder Stretch**
PAGE 30

2. **Seated Gate**
PAGE 82

3. **Seated Star**
PAGE 58

4. **Seated Leg Lift**
PAGE 88

# DYNAMIC STRETCH FLOW

**TARGETED BENEFITS:** Joint Health, Mobility and Movement

Stretch and feel the difference. This sequence is great for loosening tight muscles and increasing joint mobility, making ordinary activities easier and your overall movement more fluid. Each stretch is designed to target common problem areas—hips, hamstrings, and shoulders—releasing tension and improving range of motion. Practicing this flow regularly will improve your posture and reduce strain in your back and joints. It's ideal as a morning routine or as a cooldown after other exercise. Practice three to four times a week.

## THE SEQUENCE

1. **SEATED FORWARD FOLD WITH SHOULDER STRETCH:** Hold for 3 rounds of breath.
2. **SEATED GATE:** Hold for 3 rounds of breath.
3. **SEATED STAR:** Hold for 5 rounds of breath.
4. **SEATED LEG LIFT:** Hold for 5 rounds of breath.
5. Repeat the full sequence, switching sides with Seated Gate and Seated Leg Lift.

**Remember:** Take your time with each stretch—there's no rush! Keep your movements slow and steady and focus on breathing deeply. Let your body relax into each pose, and remember, it's okay to stop where it feels comfortable. Listen to your body—it knows best!

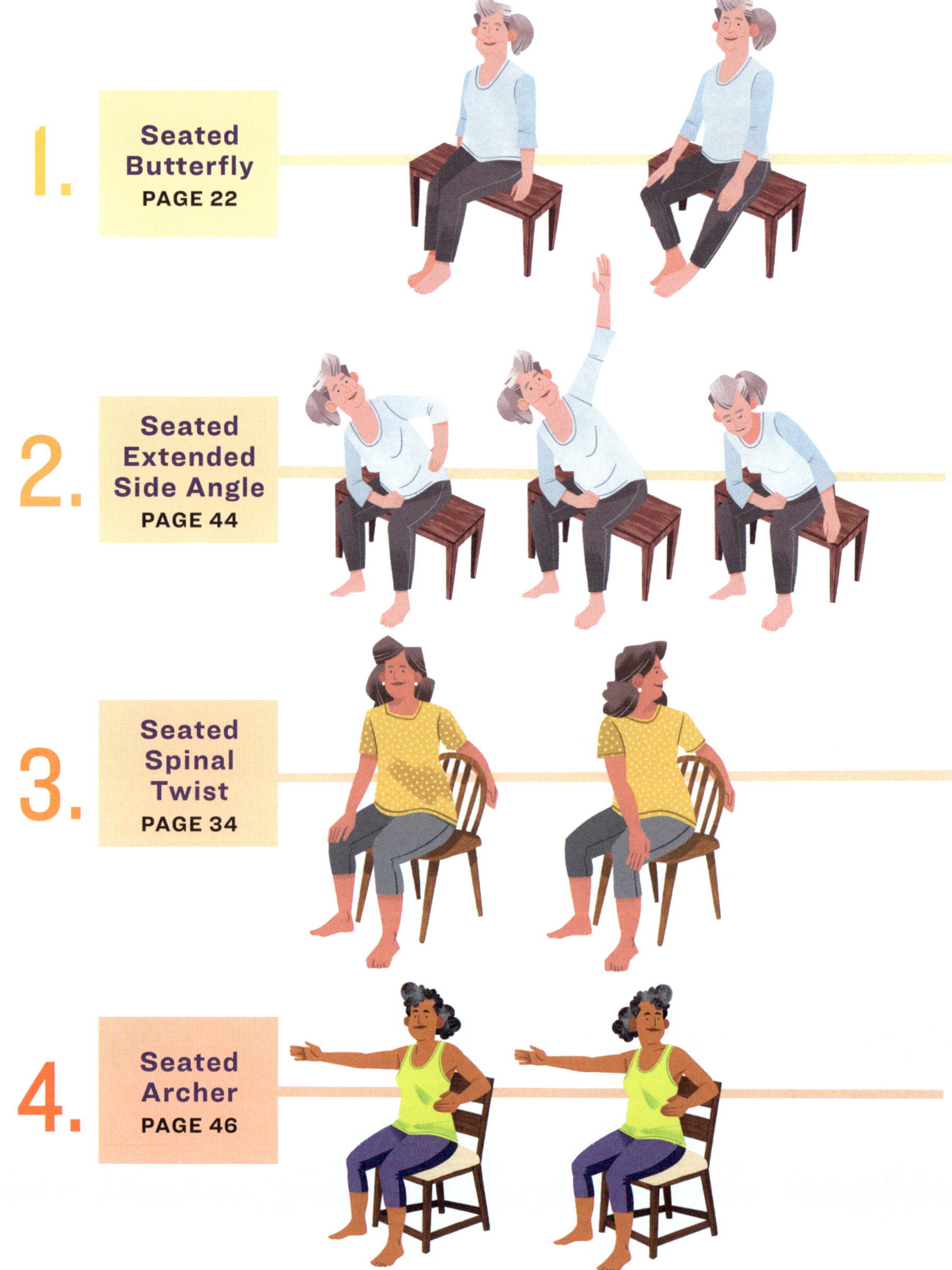
1.
Seated Butterfly
PAGE 22
2.
Seated Extended Side Angle
PAGE 44
3.
Seated Spinal Twist
PAGE 34
4.
Seated Archer
PAGE 46

# ELEGANT STRENGTH

**TARGETED BENEFITS:** Mobility and Movement, Muscle Endurance and Strength

This sequence, which emphasizes graceful, flowing movements, combines poses that target both strength-building and flexibility. The poses engage your core, legs, and arms while encouraging mindful stretching, making it a great way to improve posture and mobility. You'll notice better balance, reduced stiffness, and more control in your daily activities. This flow is perfect to wake up the body to take on the day, or as a midday boost to energize your afternoon. Aim for three times a week.

## THE SEQUENCE

1. **SEATED BUTTERFLY:** Do the open-close motion for 20 seconds or hold thighs open for three rounds of breath.
2. **SEATED EXTENDED SIDE ANGLE:** Do 3 rounds of breath on one side, then switch sides.
3. **SEATED SPINAL TWIST:** Do 3 rounds of breath on one side, then switch sides.
4. **SEATED ARCHER:** Do 3 rounds of breath on one side, then switch sides.

**Remember:** Try to move like a dancer—smooth and graceful. Keep your posture tall and your core gently engaged. Breathe deeply and let each stretch flow naturally. Focus on steady, controlled movements, and enjoy the feeling of strength and ease coming together.

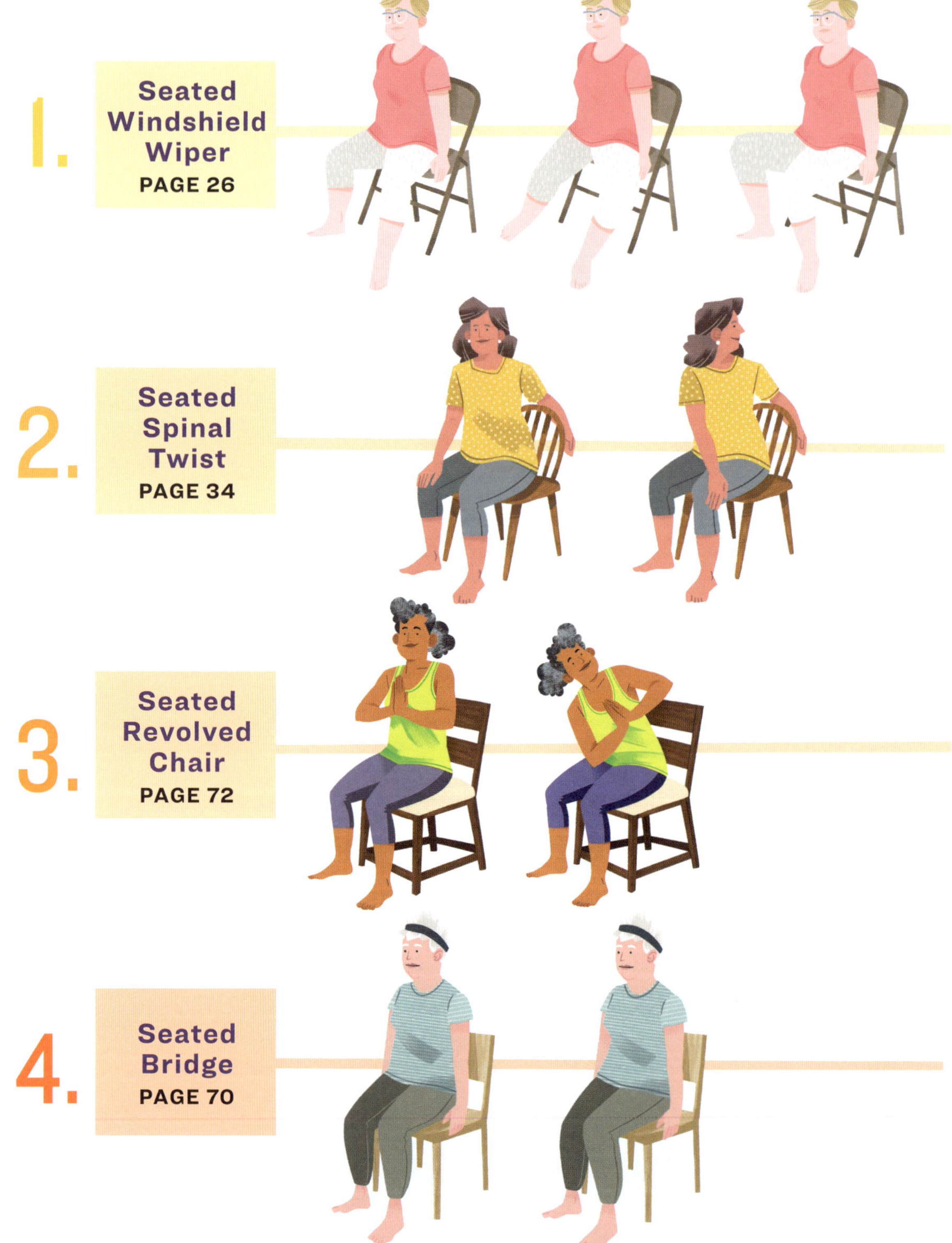
1.
Seated Windshield Wiper
PAGE 26
2.
Seated Spinal Twist
PAGE 34
3.
Seated Revolved Chair
PAGE 72
4.
Seated Bridge
PAGE 70

# GROUNDED POWER

**TARGETED BENEFITS:** Balance and Fall Prevention, Mobility and Movement

Find your power. Designed to stabilize your overall movements, this sequence strengthens your core to improve balance and posture. Practice in the morning or before a walk three to four times weekly.

## THE SEQUENCE

1. **SEATED WINDSHIELD WIPER:** Do 5 to 10 times in each direction, breathing naturally.
2. **SEATED SPINAL TWIST:** Do 3 rounds of breath.
3. **SEATED REVOLVED CHAIR:** Hold for 3 rounds of breath.
4. **SEATED BRIDGE:** Hold for 3 rounds of breath.
5. Repeat sequence, switching sides with Seated Spinal Twist and Seated Revolved Chair.

**Remember:** Sit tall and keep your movements slow and steady, focusing on balance and control. If a pose feels wobbly, that's okay! Just breathe deeply and try again—you're building strength with every practice.

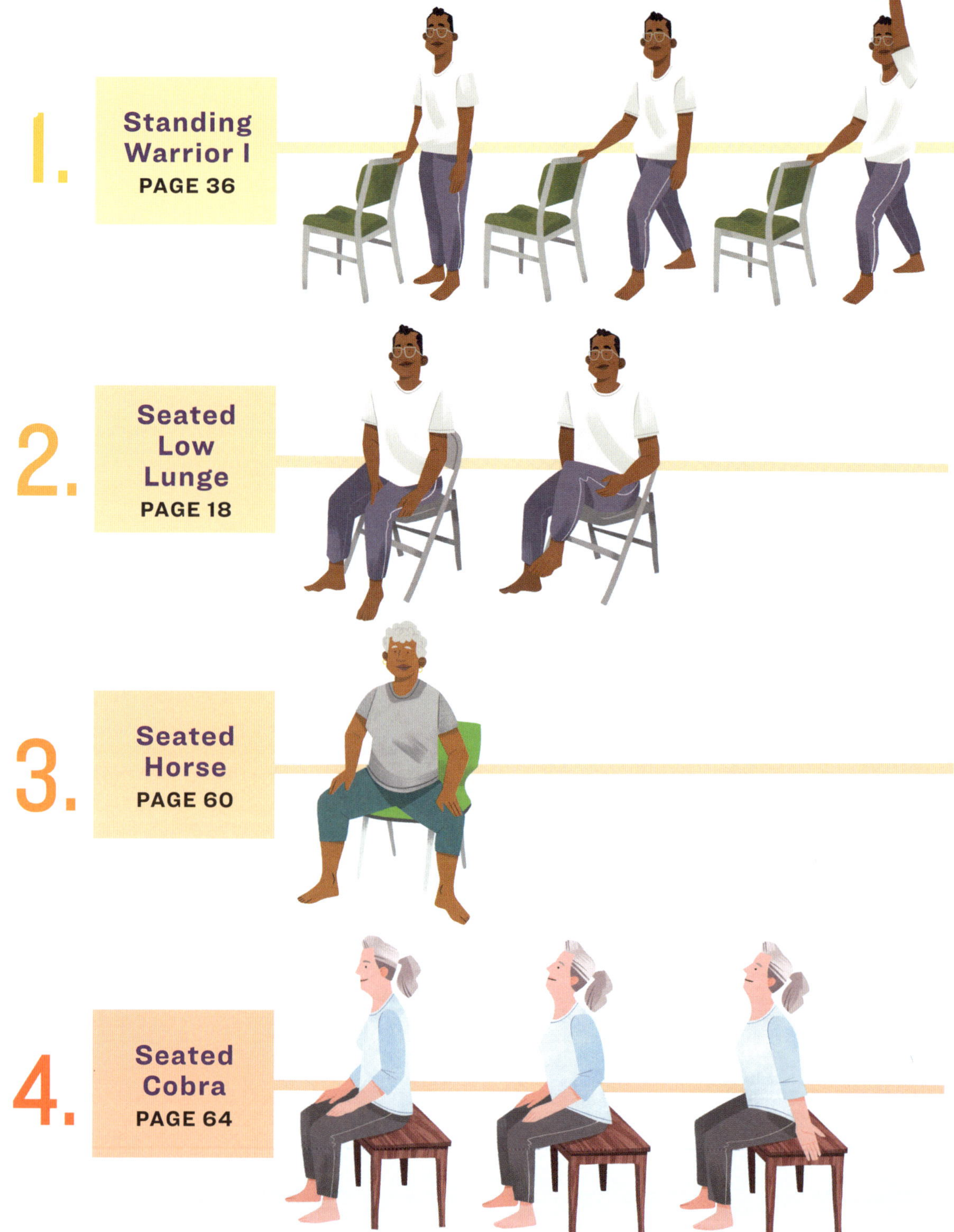
1.
Standing Warrior I
PAGE 36
2.
Seated Low Lunge
PAGE 18
3.
Seated Horse
PAGE 60
4.
Seated Cobra
PAGE 64

# LOWER-BODY FLOW

**TARGETED BENEFITS:** Joint Health, Muscle Strength and Endurance

Connect with your strength and stability. This flow focuses on your lower body, building strength and flexibility to help you stay grounded and confident in your movements. By strengthening key muscles and improving joint mobility, it makes standing, walking, and bending feel more natural. This sequence is also great for improving balance and easing stiffness after sitting for long periods, giving your body the movement it needs to feel refreshed. This sequence is ideal after sitting for a while. Practice it 3 to 4 times weekly.

## THE SEQUENCE

1. **STANDING WARRIOR I:** Hold for 3 rounds of breath.
2. **SEATED LOW LUNGE:** Repeat this pose 3 times, taking a breath between each repetition.
3. **SEATED HORSE:** Do 3 rounds of breath.
4. **SEATED COBRA:** Do 3 rounds of breath.
5. Repeat sequence, switching sides with Warrior I and Seated Low Lunge.

**Remember:** Plant your feet firmly on the ground like the roots of a tree—it'll help you feel steady and strong. Engage your legs and core as you move and breathe deeply. Take your time and feel the sense of stability and strength you're building.

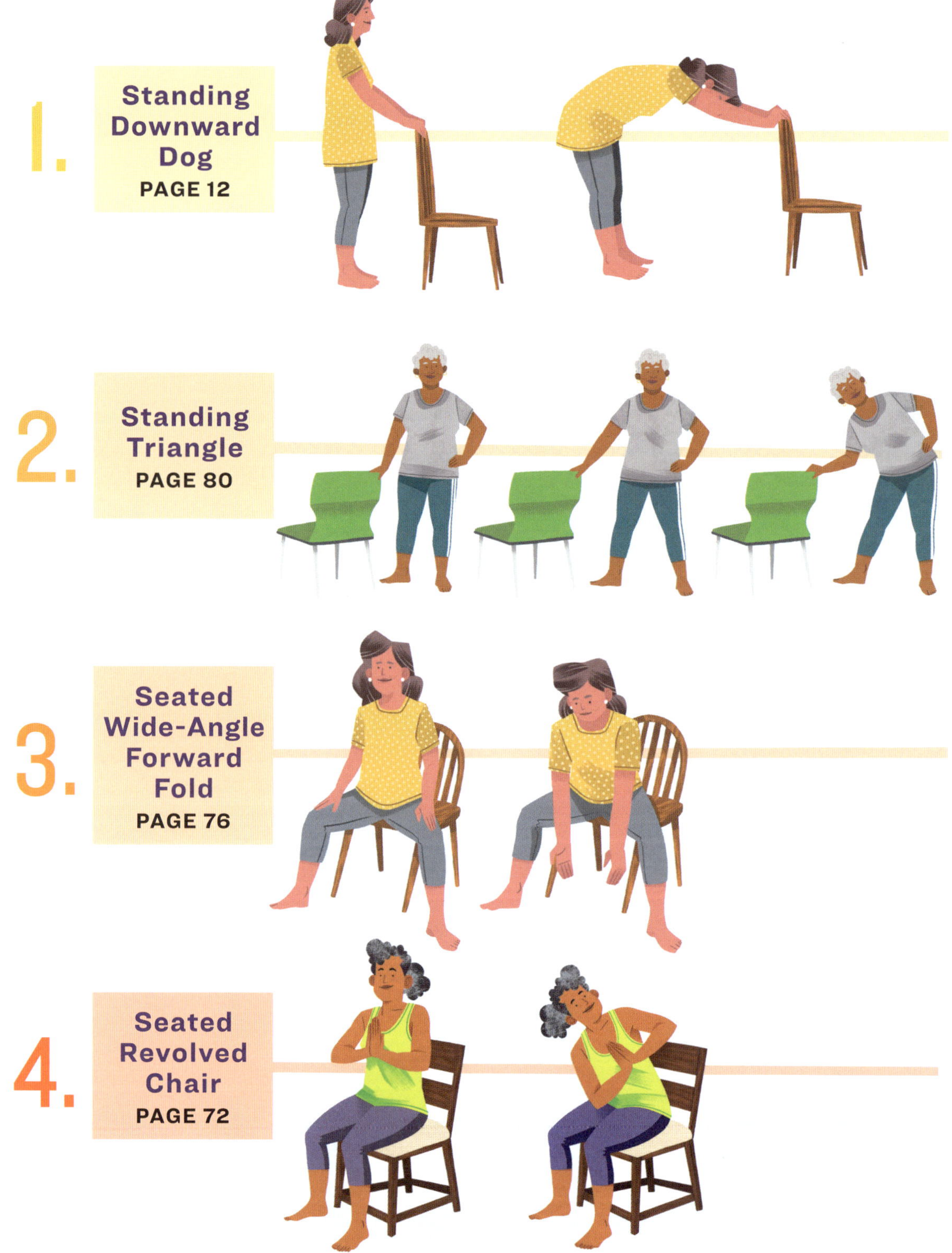
1.
Standing Downward Dog
PAGE 12
2.
Standing Triangle
PAGE 80
3.
Seated Wide-Angle Forward Fold
PAGE 76
4.
Seated Revolved Chair
PAGE 72

# FULL-BODY FLOW

**TARGETED BENEFITS:** Mobility and Movement, Muscle Endurance and Strength, Relief of Aches and Pains

Think of this flow as a gentle wake-up call for your whole body. This sequence engages your entire body, building strength and flexibility to support basic movements like reaching, lifting, and bending. Practicing this flow regularly can also help reduce stiffness and tension, promoting a sense of lightness and ease in your movements. This is great as a pre-activity warm-up. Practice three to four times weekly.

## THE SEQUENCE

1. **STANDING DOWNWARD DOG:** Hold for 3 rounds of breath.
2. **STANDING TRIANGLE:** Hold for 3 rounds of breath.
3. **SEATED WIDE-ANGLE FORWARD FOLD:** Hold for 3 rounds of breath.
4. **SEATED REVOLVED CHAIR:** Hold for 3 rounds of breath.
5. Repeat sequence, switching sides with Standing Triangle and Seated Revolved Chair.

**Remember:** After Standing Triangle, take a breath as you stand and move to sit in the chair for the next two poses. Move slowly and focus on connecting your breath with each stretch. Keep your posture tall and make sure your movements feel smooth and energized.

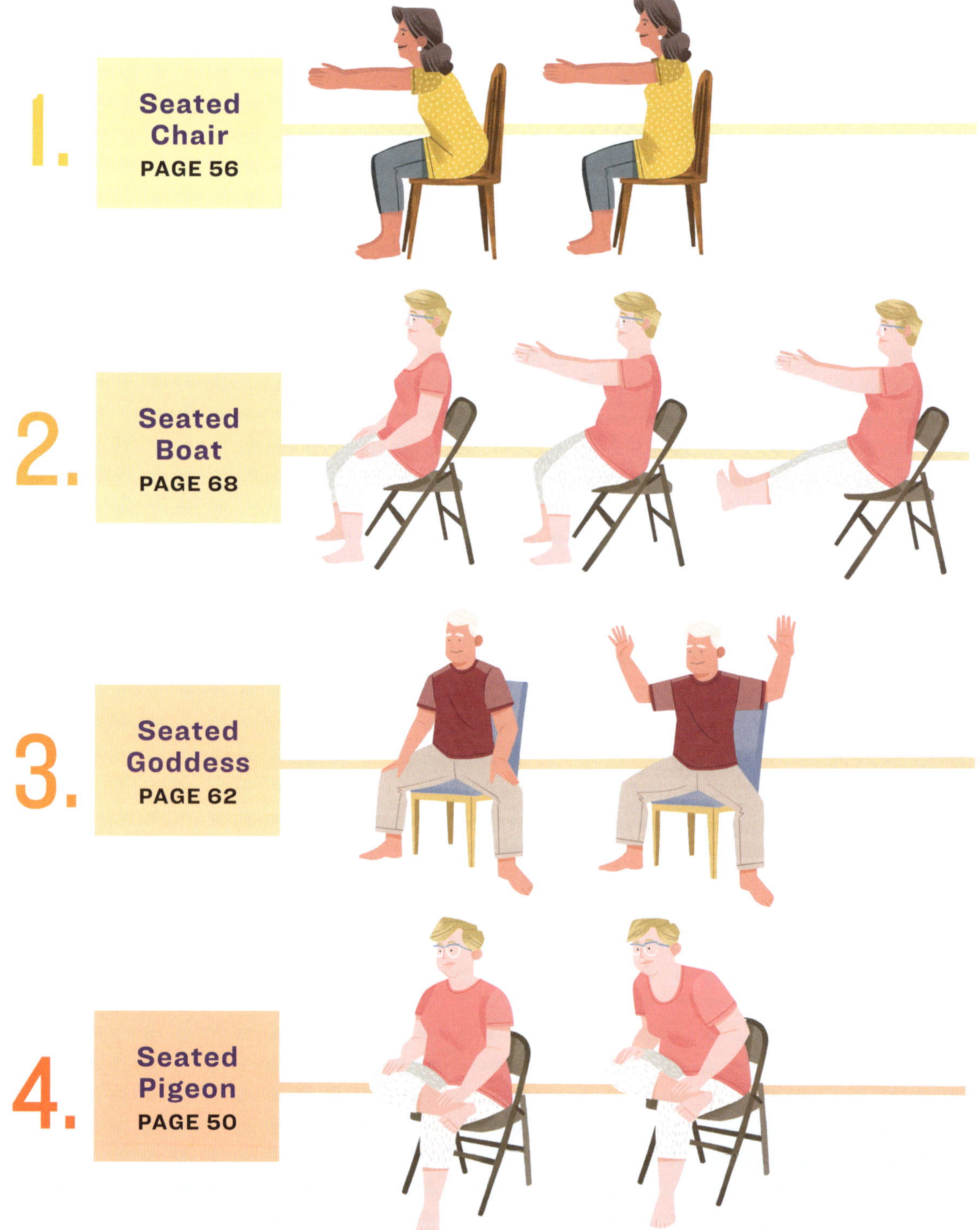
1.
Seated Chair
PAGE 56
2.
Seated Boat
PAGE 68
3.
Seated Goddess
PAGE 62
4.
Seated Pigeon
PAGE 50

# STRENGTH AND STABILITY

**TARGETED BENEFITS:** Balance and Fall Prevention, Joint Health, Muscle Strength and Endurance

Ready to feel strong, steady, and secure? This flow is designed to support better balance, posture, and coordination, making it easier to handle everyday tasks like standing, walking, and lifting. The combination of strength and stability work also reduces the risk of falls and supports joint health. Practice three to four times a week.

## THE SEQUENCE

1. **SEATED CHAIR:** Do 3 rounds of breath.
2. **SEATED BOAT:** Hold for 3 rounds of breath.
3. **SEATED GODDESS:** Do 3 rounds of breath.
4. **SEATED PIGEON:** Do 3 rounds of breath, then switch legs and repeat.

**Remember:** Focus on feeling steady in each pose before moving to the next. Engage your core and press firmly through your feet for balance. Remember, it's not about speed, it's about building strength with every movement.

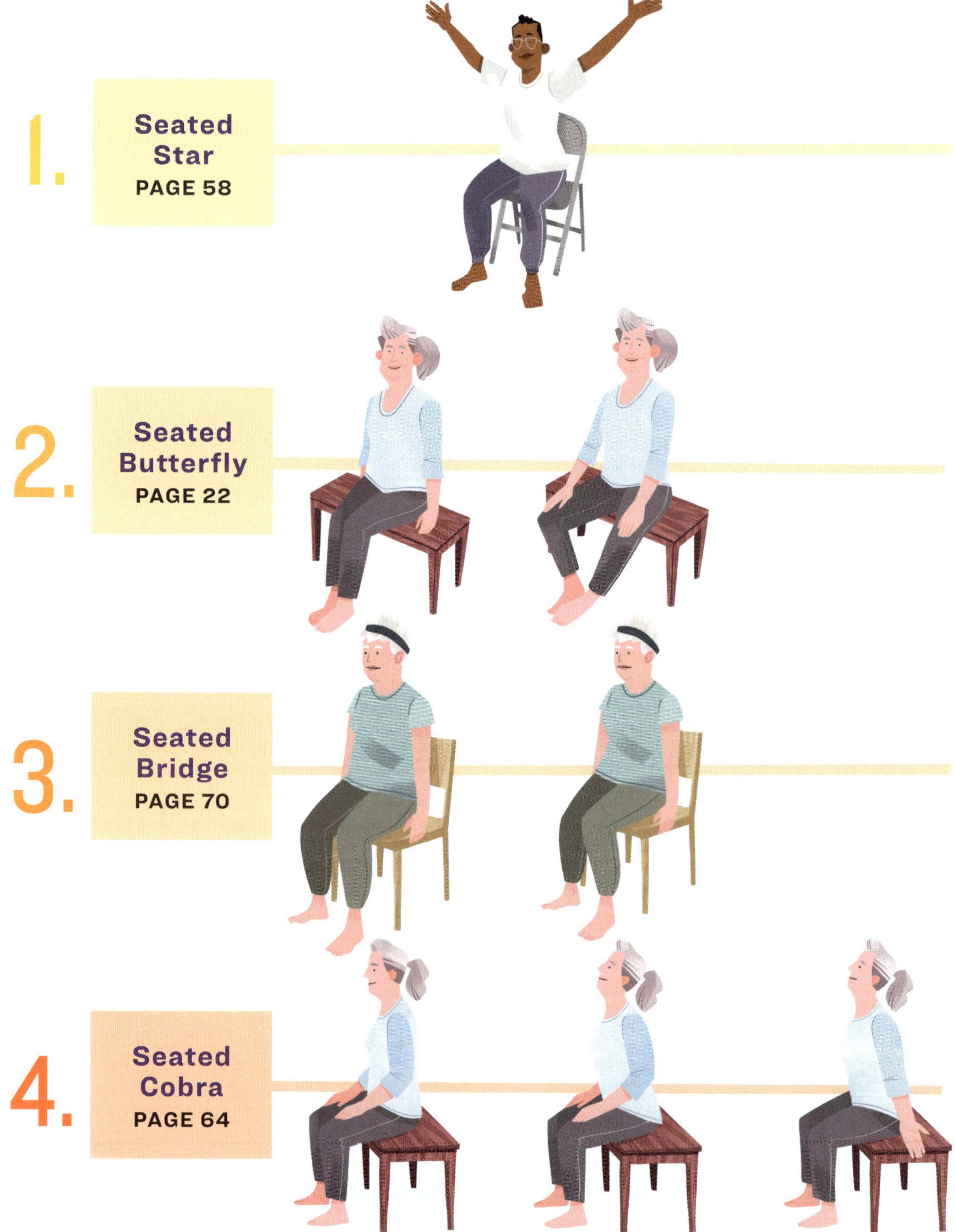
1.
Seated Star
PAGE 58
2.
Seated Butterfly
PAGE 22
3.
Seated Bridge
PAGE 70
4.
Seated Cobra
PAGE 64

# RELAXED POWER

**TARGETED BENEFITS:** Joint Health, Mobility and Movement, Relief of Aches and Pains

This calming sequence combines gentle stretches and strength-building poses to help you release tension and recharge. It's perfect for improving flexibility and joint health while promoting mindfulness and focus. The soothing movements also encourage deep breathing, which helps reduce stress and improve circulation. This sequence is ideal after exercise or as a relaxing evening practice. Do it three times a week.

## THE SEQUENCE

1. **SEATED STAR:** Do 5 rounds of breath.
2. **SEATED BUTTERFLY:** Do 10 repetitions, or hold the pose for 3 to 5 rounds of breath.
3. **SEATED BRIDGE:** Hold for 3 to 5 rounds of breath.
4. **SEATED COBRA:** Do 3 rounds of breath.

**Remember:** Think of this sequence as your chance to unwind and recharge. Move slowly, focusing on each muscle group as you go. Stay present, breathe deeply, and enjoy the feeling of releasing tension while building gentle strength.

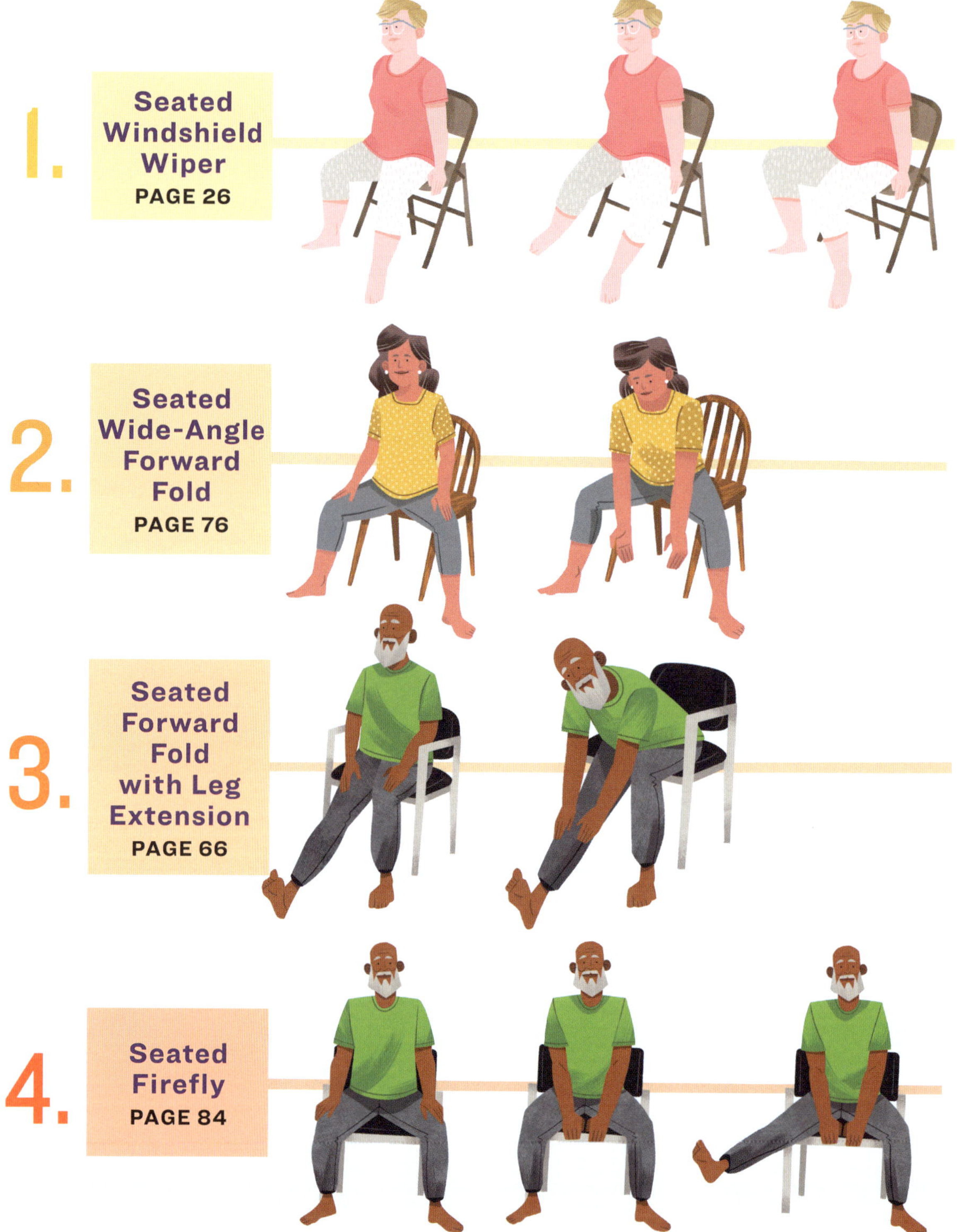
1.
Seated Windshield Wiper
PAGE 26
2.
Seated Wide-Angle Forward Fold
PAGE 76
3.
Seated Forward Fold with Leg Extension
PAGE 66
4.
Seated Firefly
PAGE 84

# HIPS AND HAMSTRINGS

**TARGETED BENEFITS:** Joint Health, Mobility and Movement, Relief of Aches and Pains

Stretch away stiffness. Loosen tight hips and stretch your hamstrings with this simple flow that starts with movement. It's great for reducing stiffness and discomfort in ordinary movement, and makes the occasional bend, long walk, and prolonged period of sitting more comfortable. The poses also support better posture and alignment, easing strain on your back and knees. Perform this sequence after a walk or during the day to release tightness. Practice three times weekly.

## THE SEQUENCE

1. **SEATED WINDSHIELD WIPER:** Do 10 times in each direction, breathing naturally.
2. **SEATED WIDE-ANGLE FORWARD FOLD:** Hold for 3 rounds of breath and repeat on the other side.
3. **SEATED FORWARD FOLD WITH LEG EXTENSION:** Hold for 3 rounds of breath and repeat on the other side.
4. **SEATED FIREFLY:** Hold for 3 rounds of breath. If lifting one leg, repeat on the other side.

**Remember:** Let your breath guide each stretch. Keep your back straight as you hinge forward, and don't reach farther than feels natural. With each pose, imagine the tension melting away from your hips and legs, leaving you feeling lighter and more mobile.

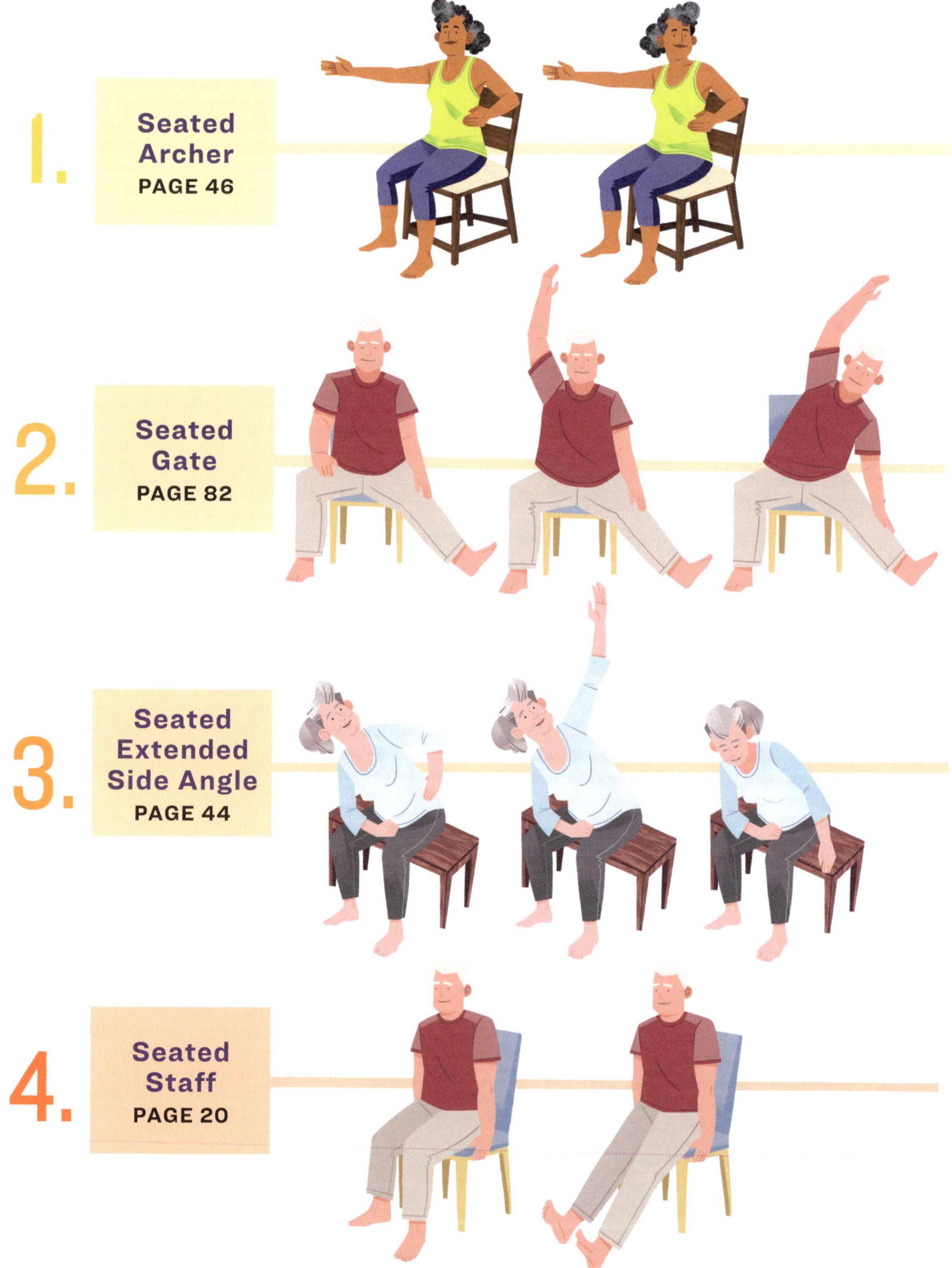
1.
Seated Archer
PAGE 46
2.
Seated Gate
PAGE 82
3.
Seated Extended Side Angle
PAGE 44
4.
Seated Staff
PAGE 20

# FLOWING FOCUS

**TARGETED BENEFITS:** Mobility and Movement, Overall Well-Being, Relief of Aches and Pains

This flow is perfect for reconnecting with your body and calming your mind while supporting better mobility. The flowing movements help you loosen tight muscles and reduce stiffness, making it easier to move through your day with ease. Over time, you'll notice smoother, more fluid movements that will help you feel energized and ready to take on whatever comes your way. It's great as a morning starter or a refreshing break during your day. Practice three to four times weekly.

## THE SEQUENCE

1. **SEATED ARCHER:** Do 3 rounds of breath.
2. **SEATED GATE:** Do 3 rounds of breath.
3. **SEATED EXTENDED SIDE ANGLE:** Do 3 rounds of breath.
4. **SEATED STAFF:** Do 3 rounds of breath.
5. Repeat full sequence, switching sides on Seated Archer, Seated Gate, Seated Extended Side Angle, and Seated Staff.

**Remember:** Think of this flow as a gentle wave—move smoothly from one pose to the next. Keep your core engaged and your feet firmly grounded to maintain balance. Let your breath guide the transition for a calm and steady flow.

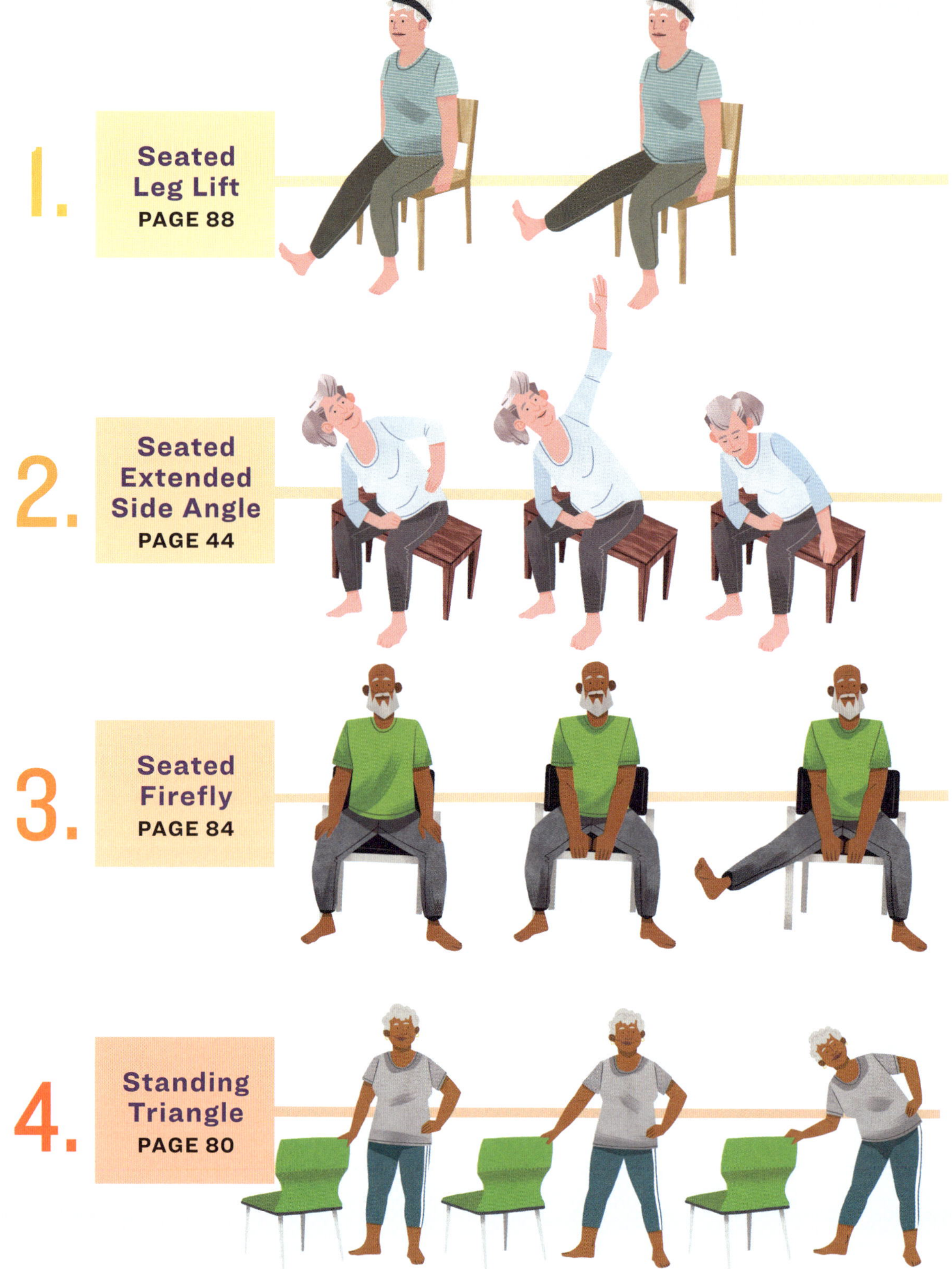
1.
Seated Leg Lift
PAGE 88
2.
Seated Extended Side Angle
PAGE 44
3.
Seated Firefly
PAGE 84
4.
Standing Triangle
PAGE 80

# STABLE STRENGTH

**TARGETED BENEFITS:** Joint Health, Muscle Endurance and Strength

Build strong legs and stay steady. This flow also helps maintain muscle mass and bone health. With practice, you'll notice greater endurance and control in everyday activities. This sequence is ideal for activating your legs. Try it three times a week.

## THE SEQUENCE

1. **SEATED LEG LIFT:** Do 3 times.
2. **SEATED EXTENDED SIDE ANGLE:** Do 3 rounds of breath.
3. **SEATED FIREFLY:** Do 3 rounds of breath.
4. **STANDING TRIANGLE:** Do 3 rounds of breath.
5. Repeat the sequence, switching sides with Seated Leg Lift, Seated Extended Side Angle, and Standing Triangle.

**Remember:** Focus on pressing firmly through your feet and engaging your thighs in each pose. As you move, keep your posture tall and your core gently activated for extra support.

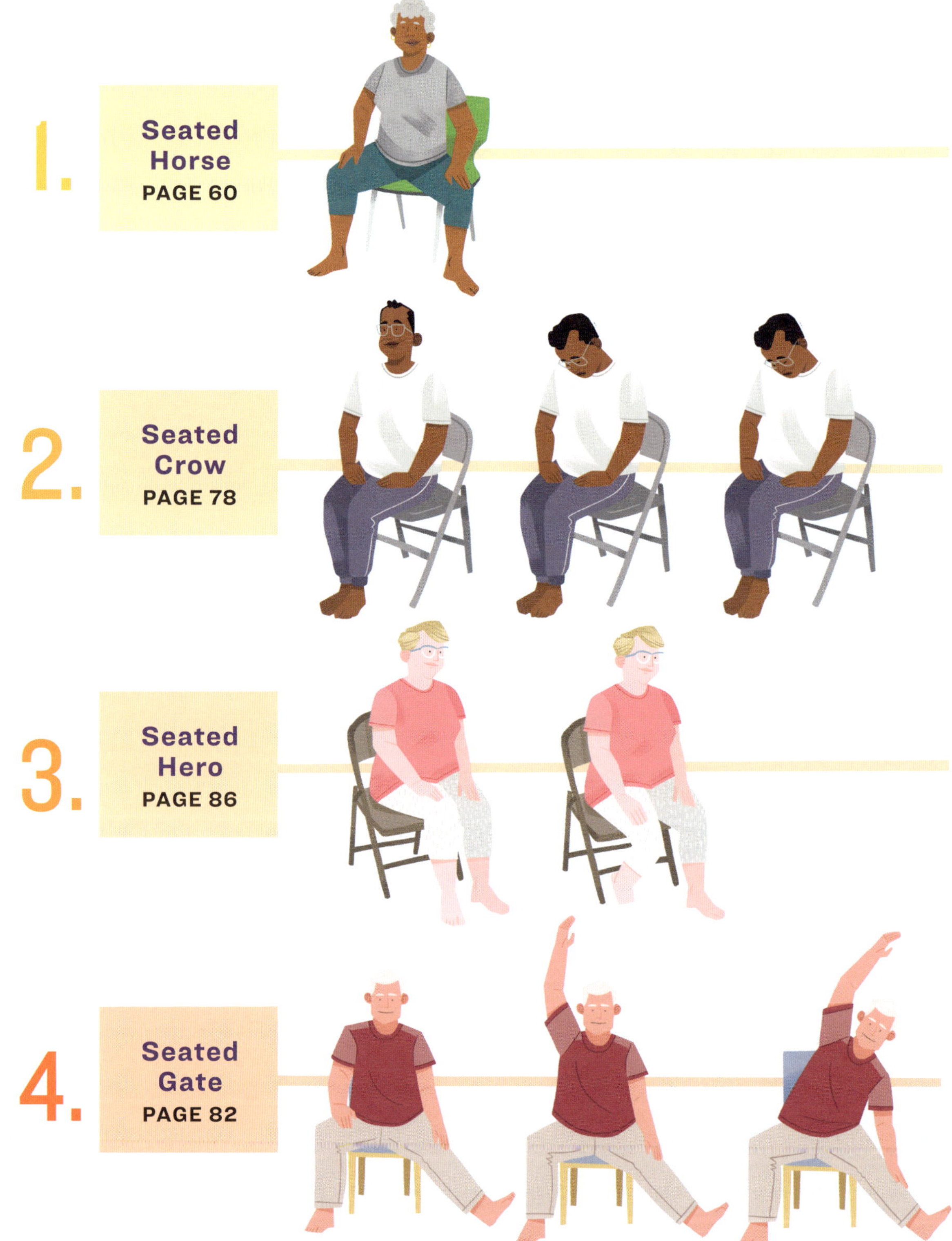
1.
Seated
Horse
PAGE 60
2.
Seated
Crow
PAGE 78
3.
Seated
Hero
PAGE 86
4.
Seated
Gate
PAGE 82

# GROUNDED MOBILITY FLOW

**TARGETED BENEFITS:** Balance and Fall Prevention, Joint Health, Mobility and Movement

These poses work to reduce stiffness and support smooth movements. You'll also notice better balance, making everyday tasks like handling steps or standing up from a chair more effortless. Try this flow as part of a lower-body workout. Practice 3 times weekly.

## THE SEQUENCE

1. **SEATED HORSE:** Do 3 rounds of breath.
2. **SEATED CROW:** Do 3 rounds of breath.
3. **SEATED HERO:** Hold for 3 rounds of breath.
4. **SEATED GATE:** Do 3 rounds of breath.
5. Repeat sequence and switch sides with Seated Horse and Seated Gate.

**Remember:** Keep your back straight and shoulders relaxed, and let your breath guide each pose.

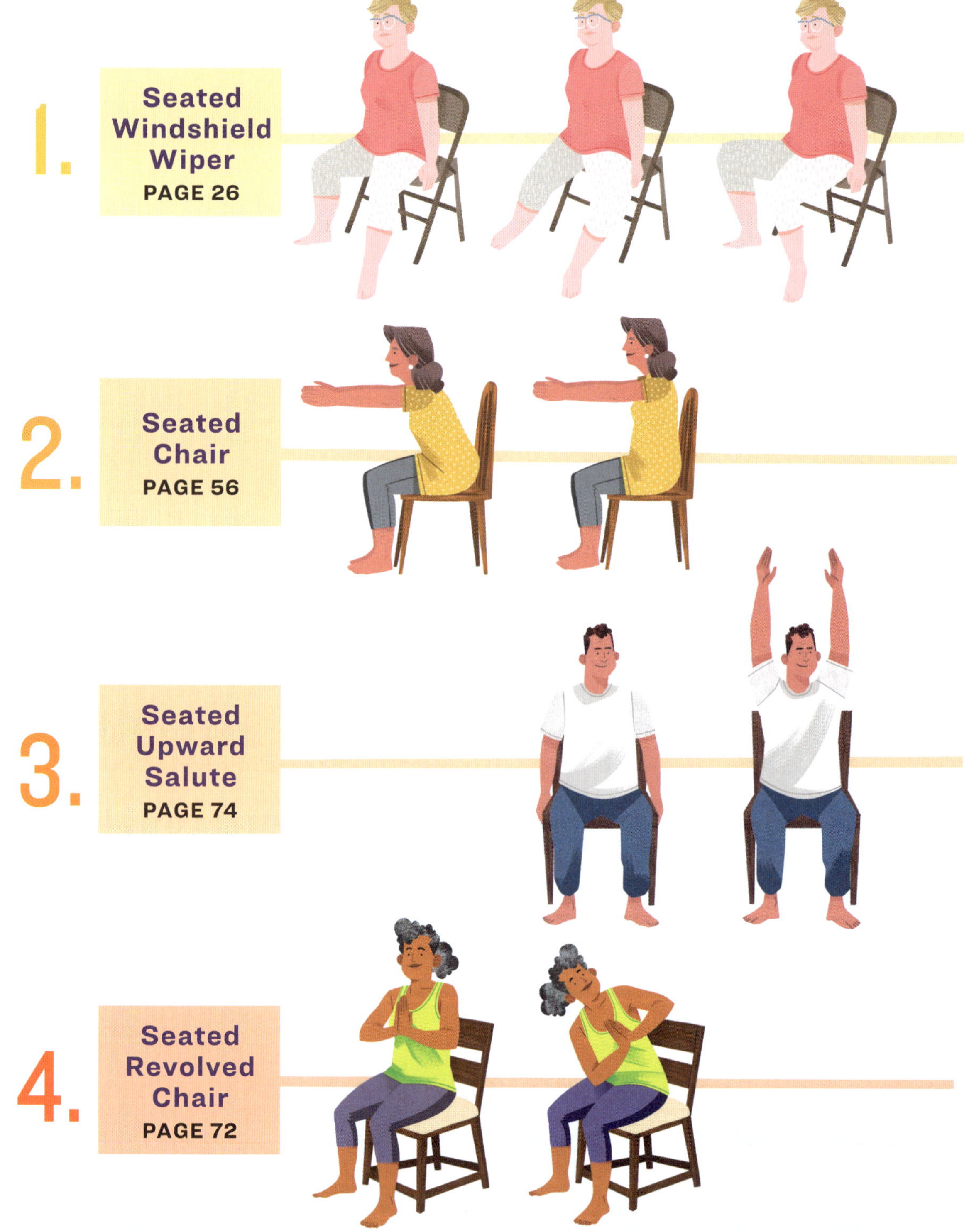
1.
Seated Windshield Wiper
PAGE 26
2.
Seated Chair
PAGE 56
3.
Seated Upward Salute
PAGE 74
4.
Seated Revolved Chair
PAGE 72

# CORE AND MORE FLOW

**TARGETED BENEFITS:** Balance and Fall Prevention, Mobility and Movement

I always love when I can target different muscle groups in a workout. This flow gently moves from warming up your core and lower body to strengthening, stretching, and finally a twisting movement to release tension. Use this sequence three times per week, especially as a morning core activator.

## THE SEQUENCE

1. **WINDSHIELD WIPER:** Do 10 times in each direction, breathing naturally.
2. **SEATED CHAIR:** Do 3 rounds of breath.
3. **SEATED UPWARD SALUTE:** Hold for 3 rounds of breath.
4. **SEATED REVOLVED CHAIR:** Hold for 3 rounds of breath.
5. Repeat full sequence, switching sides with Seated Upward Salute Pose and Seated Revolved Chair Pose.

**Remember:** Imagine your belly button gently pulling toward your spine for extra stability. If you feel shaky, that's okay—you're building strength to stabilize your body.

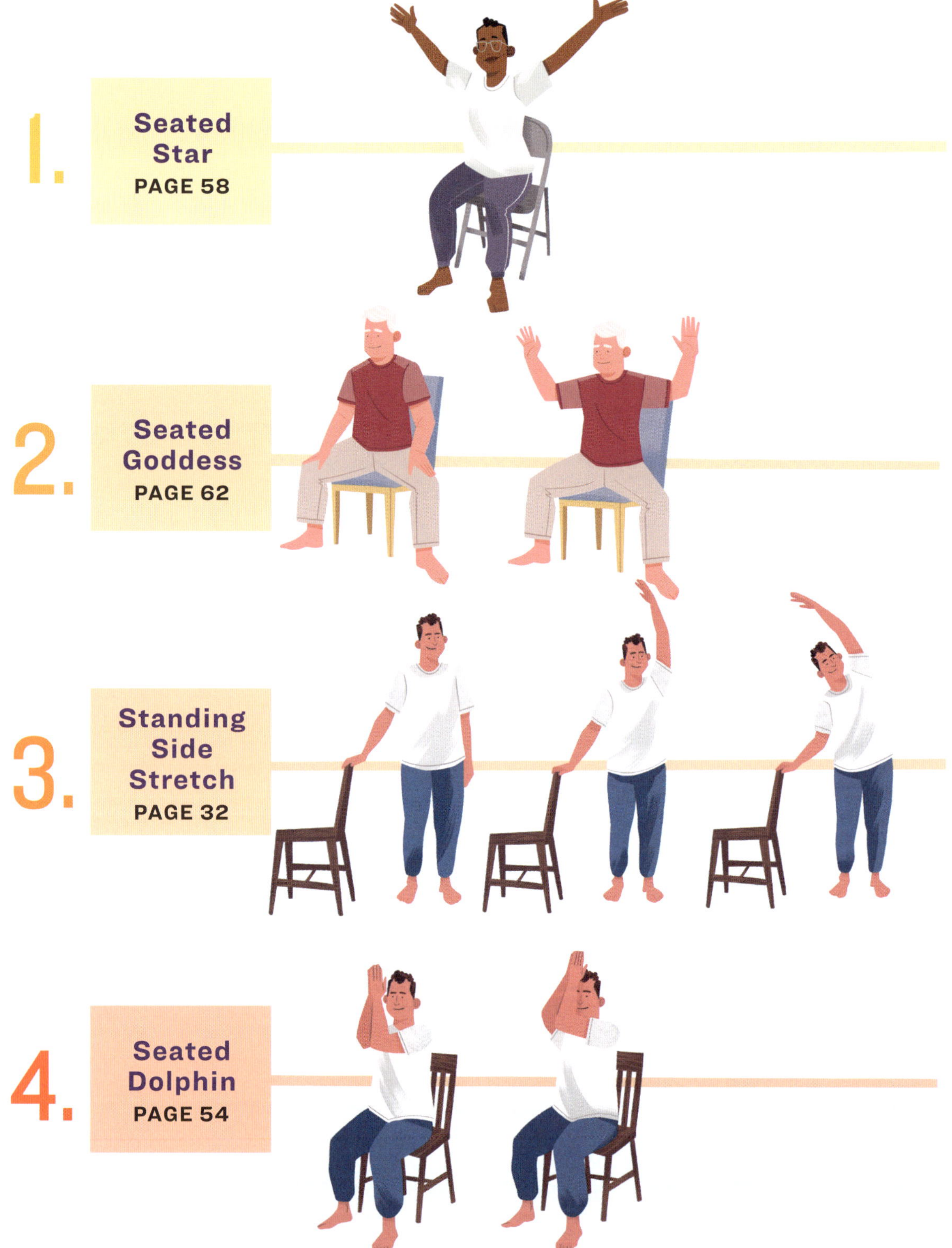
1.
Seated
Star
PAGE 58
2.
Seated
Goddess
PAGE 62
3.
Standing
Side
Stretch
PAGE 32
4.
Seated
Dolphin
PAGE 54

# RISING STAR

**TARGETED BENEFITS:** Mobility and Movement, Overall Well-Being, Relief of Aches and Pains

This sequence is designed to uplift, restore, and empower—leaving you feeling aligned, open, and strong. Starting with Seated Star will open your body and mind before flowing into deep stretches and activating your shoulders, back, and arms. Reach for the stars three times or more a week to build your posture and flexibility

## THE SEQUENCE

1. **SEATED STAR:** Hold for 5 rounds of breath.
2. **SEATED GODDESS:** Hold for 3 rounds of breath.
3. **SEATED SIDE STRETCH:** Hold for 5 rounds of breath and switch sides.
4. **SEATED DOLPHIN:** Hold for 3 rounds of breath.

**Remember:** Sit tall and lengthen your spine through this sequence to flow smoothly from one pose to the next.

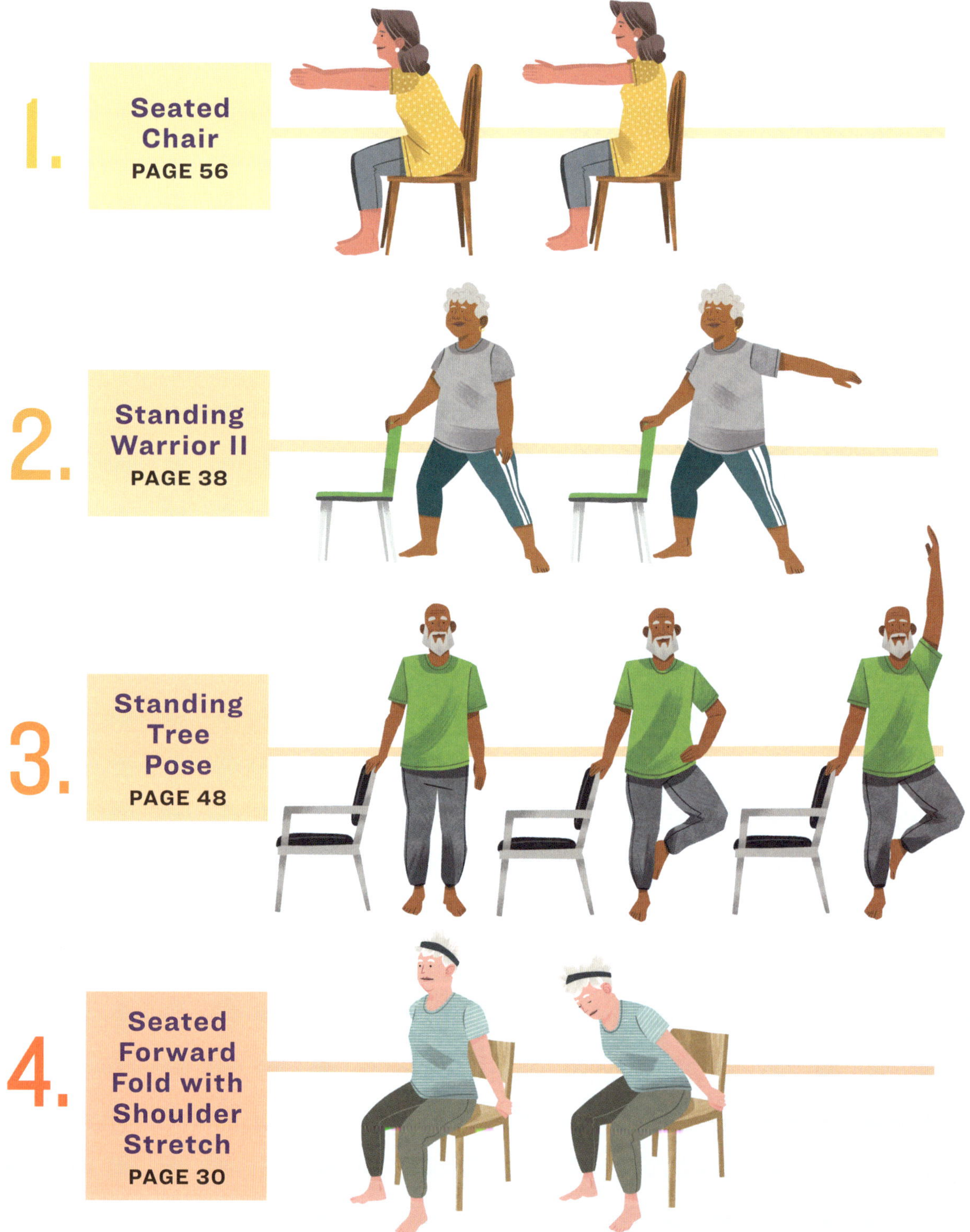

1.
Seated
Chair
PAGE 56
2.
Standing
Warrior II
PAGE 38
3.
Standing
Tree
Pose
PAGE 48
4.
Seated
Forward
Fold with
Shoulder
Stretch
PAGE 30

# STRENGTH AND STRETCH FLOW

**TARGETED BENEFITS:** Joint Health, Mobility and Movement, Muscle Endurance and Strength

I like this sequence because it's superefficient—it releases tension and strengthens my muscles, which is especially helpful during a busy day working on the computer. With this sequence, you'll improve flexibility and build strength, helping you move easily throughout your day. An added benefit is that it helps improve posture. It's perfect for a midmorning or post-activity routine. Practice it three times a week.

## THE SEQUENCE

1. **SEATED CHAIR:** Do 3 rounds of breath.
2. **STANDING WARRIOR II:** Do 3 rounds of breath.
3. **STANDING TREE:** Do 3 rounds of breath.
4. **SEATED FORWARD FOLD WITH SHOULDER STRETCH:** Hold for 3 rounds of breath.
5. Repeat full sequence, switching sides with Standing Warrior II and Standing Tree.

**Remember:** Think of this sequence as a blend of power and ease. Focus on engaging your muscles during the poses and relaxing deeply into each. Keep your movements smooth and steady. Return to Seated Mountain (page 10) as a transition between Standing Tree and Seated Forward Fold with Shoulder Stretch.

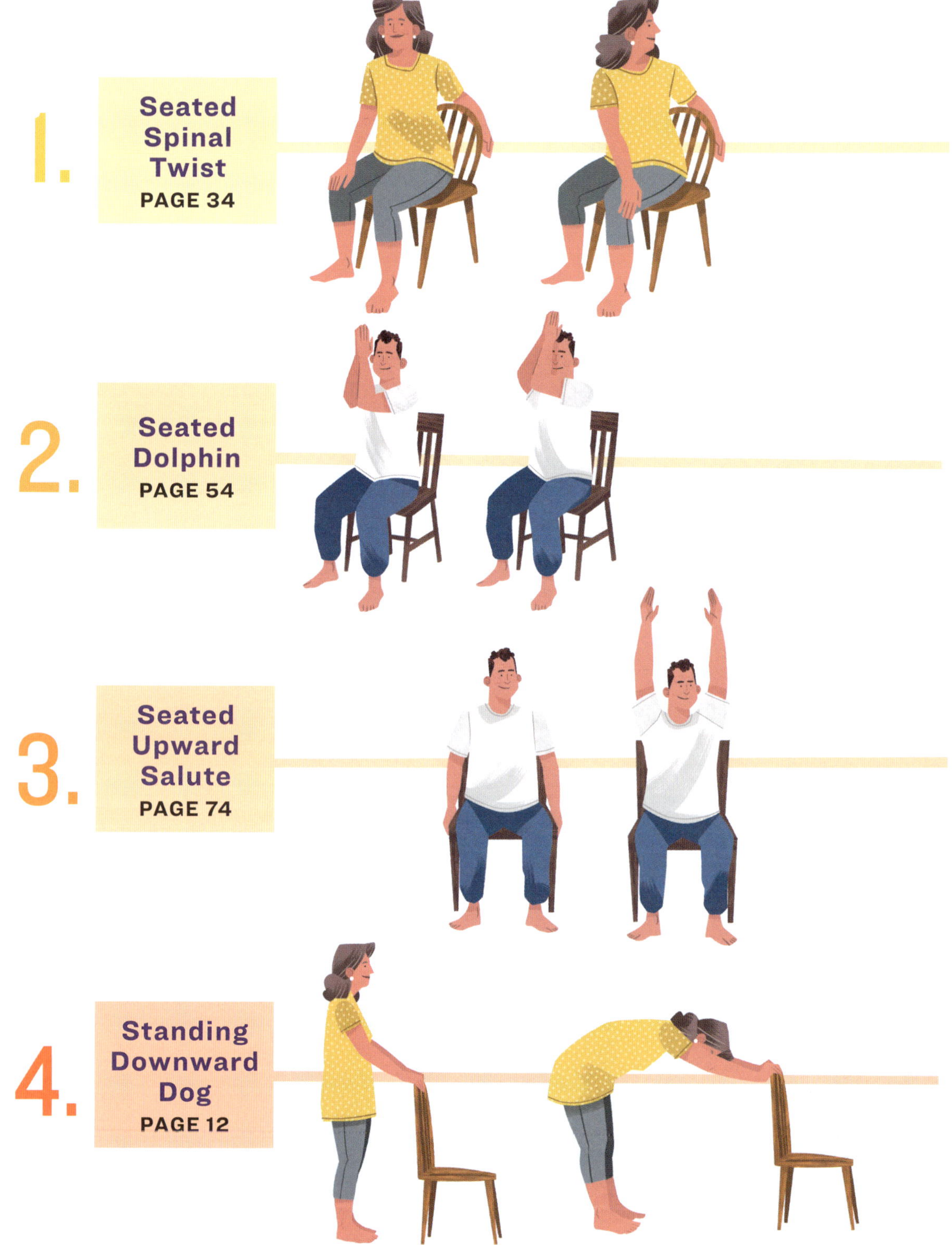
1.
Seated Spinal Twist
PAGE 34
2.
Seated Dolphin
PAGE 54
3.
Seated Upward Salute
PAGE 74
4.
Standing Downward Dog
PAGE 12

# POSTURE ENHANCER

**TARGETED BENEFITS:** Balance and Fall Prevention, Mobility and Movement

This flow strengthens and stretches the muscles that help you sit or stand upright. Good posture promotes proper alignment of your muscles and joints, ensuring everything moves effectively and efficiently. Start off your day with this flow or try it during the day for a boost. Practice three times weekly.

## THE SEQUENCE

1. **SEATED SPINAL TWIST:** Hold for 3 rounds of breath and switch sides.
2. **SEATED DOLPHIN:** Hold for 3 rounds of breath.
3. **SEATED UPWARD SALUTE:** Hold for 3 rounds of breath
4. **STANDING DOWNWARD DOG:** Hold for 3 rounds of breath.

**Remember:** Stay focused with your feet firmly planted on the floor in the seated and standing positions. Imagine your core as your anchor, keeping you steady.

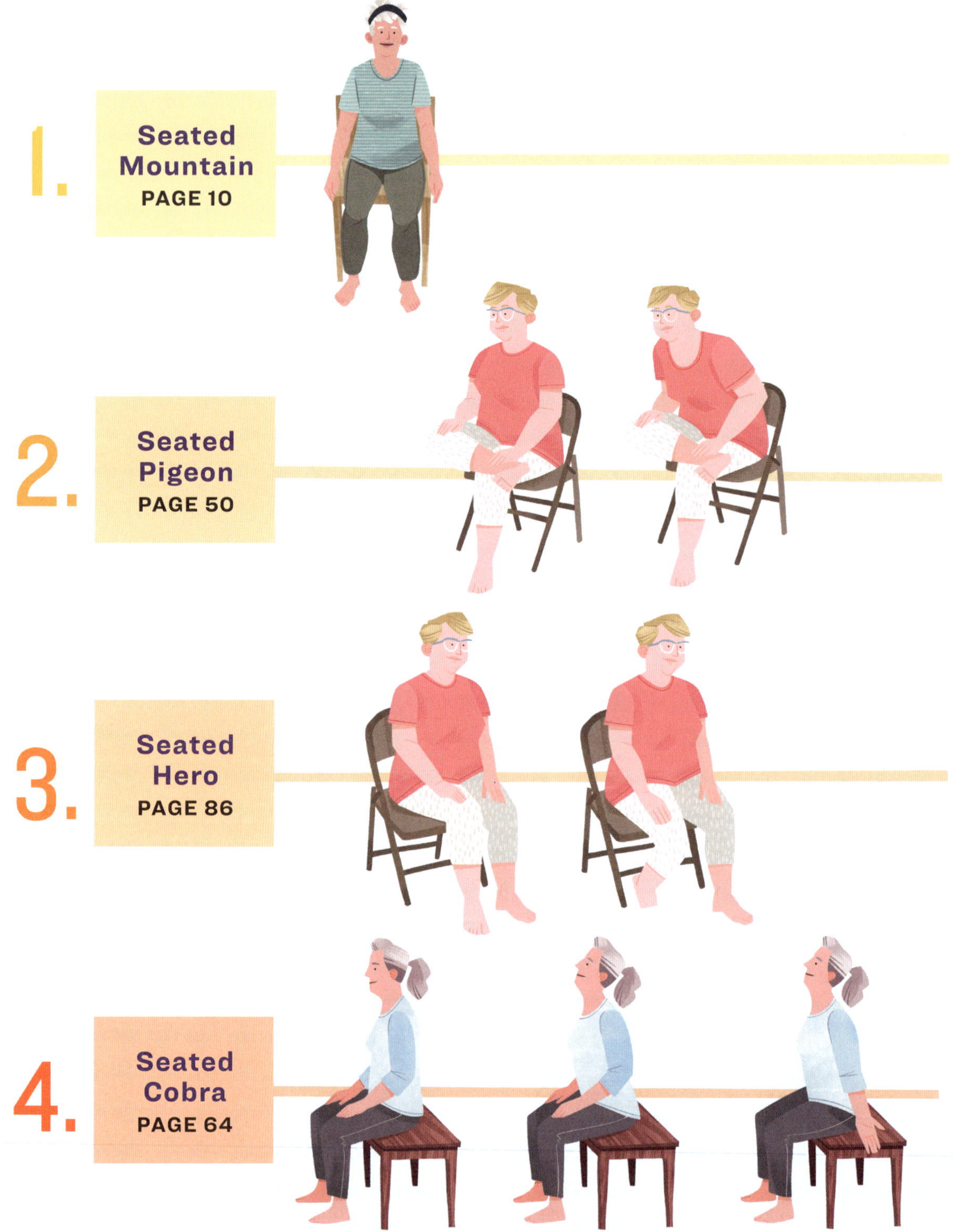
1.
Seated
Mountain
PAGE 10
2.
Seated
Pigeon
PAGE 50
3.
Seated
Hero
PAGE 86
4.
Seated
Cobra
PAGE 64

# RELAXATION AND FOCUS

**TARGETED BENEFITS:** Joint Health, Relief of Aches and Pains

Unwind your body and calm your mind. Whether you've had a busy day or just want to take a moment for yourself, this sequence will leave you feeling calm and refreshed. Ideal for relaxation in the evening or after exercise. Practice this sequence three to four times weekly.

## THE SEQUENCE

1. **SEATED MOUNTAIN:** Do 3 rounds of breath.
2. **SEATED PIGEON:** Hold for 3 rounds of breath and switch sides.
3. **SEATED HERO:** Do 3 rounds of breath.
4. **SEATED COBRA:** Hold for 3 rounds of breath.

**Remember:** Close your eyes if it feels comfortable and focus on your breath. Let go of any tension as you move gently through the poses.

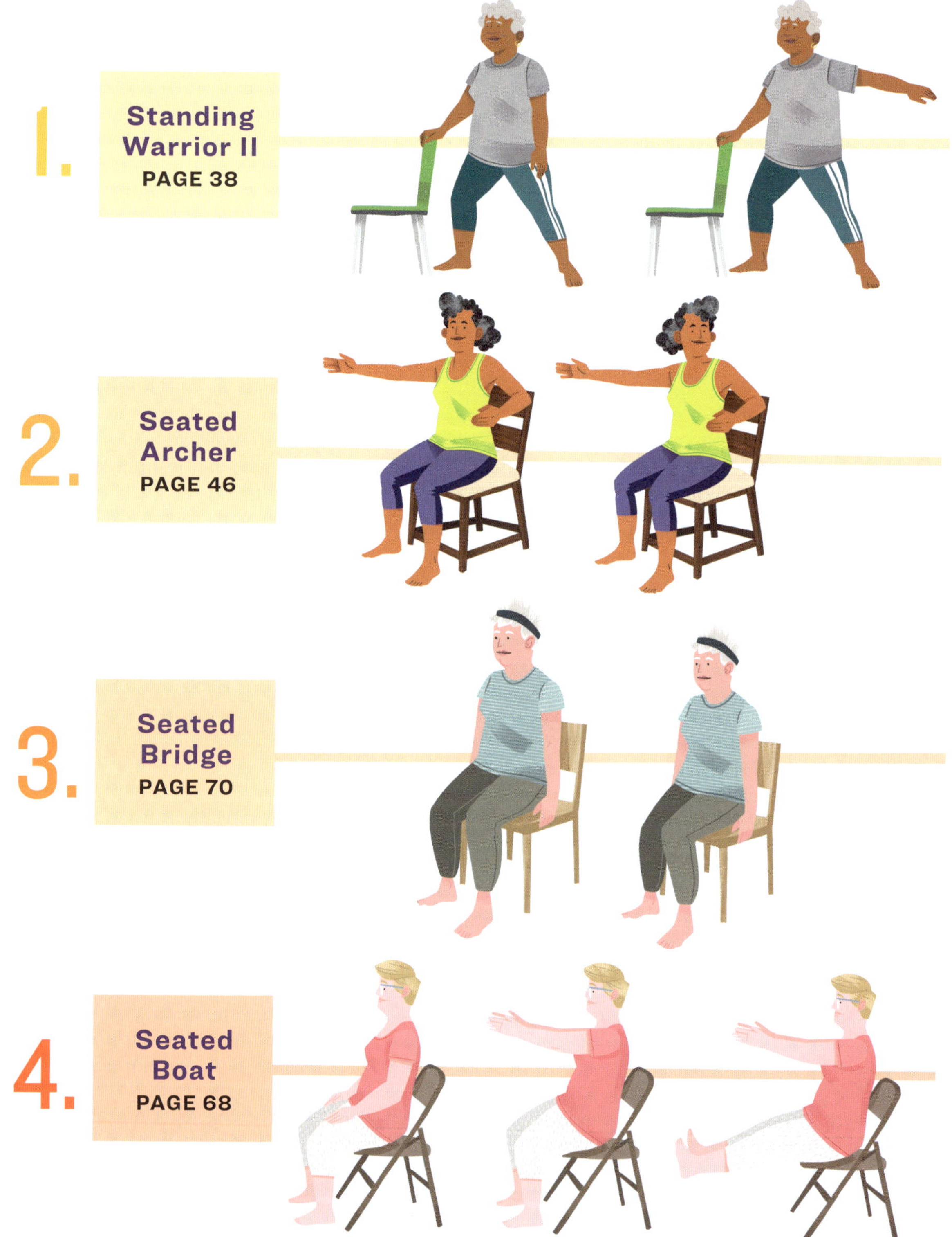

1.
Standing Warrior II
PAGE 38
2.
Seated Archer
PAGE 46
3.
Seated Bridge
PAGE 70
4.
Seated Boat
PAGE 68

# VICTORY VOYAGE

**TARGETED BENEFITS:** Balance and Fall Prevention, Muscle Endurance and Strength

With the heart of a warrior and precision of an archer, claim your victory over improved strength and balance with this powerful flow. This flow will improve stability and control, whether you're lifting objects or simply standing tall. This sequence is great to kick off your day or as part of a strength session. Practice it three to four times a week.

## THE SEQUENCE

1. **STANDING WARRIOR II:** Do 5 rounds of breath and switch sides.
2. **SEATED ARCHER:** Do 5 rounds of breath and switch sides.
3. **SEATED BRIDGE:** Hold for 3 rounds of breath.
4. **SEATED BOAT:** Hold for 20 seconds, or 3 rounds of breath.
5. Repeat sequence.

**Remember:** Focus on staying steady and strong in each pose—press through your feet and engage your core to feel grounded. Use Seated Mountain (page 10) as a transition between Standing Warrior II and Seated Archer.

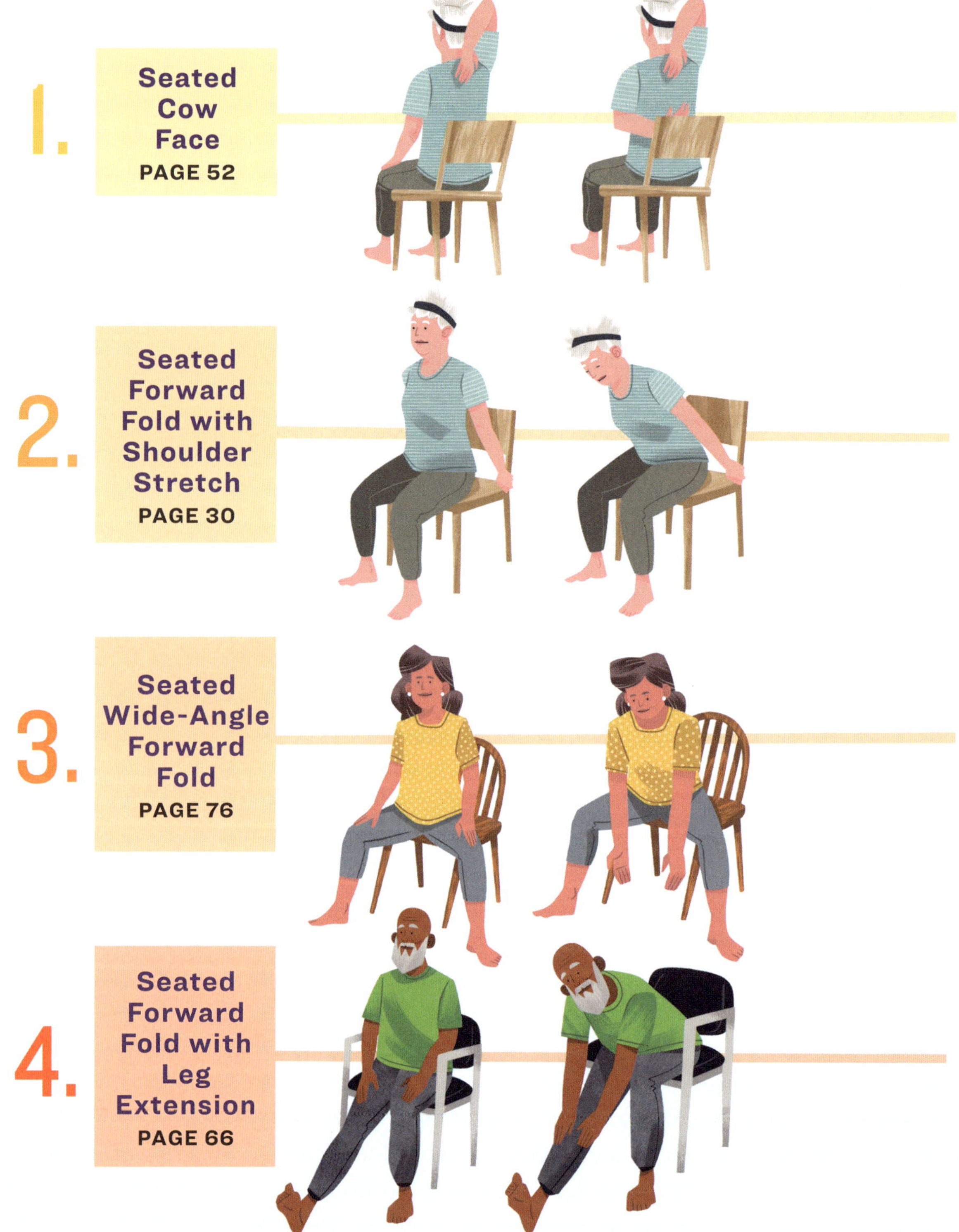
1.
Seated Cow Face
PAGE 52
2.
Seated Forward Fold with Shoulder Stretch
PAGE 30
3.
Seated Wide-Angle Forward Fold
PAGE 76
4.
Seated Forward Fold with Leg Extension
PAGE 66

# POWERFUL STRETCH FLOW

**TARGETED BENEFITS:** Joint Health, Mobility and Movement

Stretch away tension and feel flexible. This full-body flow helps loosen tight muscles and improve your range of motion by reducing stiffness and strain all over your body. Use this sequence at the start of your day, after exercise, or in the evening to relax. Practice three times weekly.

## THE SEQUENCE

1. **SEATED COW FACE:** Hold for 3 rounds of breath.
2. **SEATED FORWARD FOLD WITH SHOULDER STRETCH:** Hold for 5 rounds of breath.
3. **SEATED WIDE-ANGLE FORWARD FOLD:** Hold for 5 rounds of breath.
4. **SEATED FORWARD FOLD WITH LEG EXTENSION:** Hold for 5 rounds of breath.
5. Repeat sequence, switching sides with Seated Cow Face and Seated Forward Fold with Leg Extension.

**Remember:** Think of each stretch as a way to create space in your body. Focus on lengthening through your spine and reaching gently without forcing. Breathe deeply and let the stretches feel relaxing and refreshing.

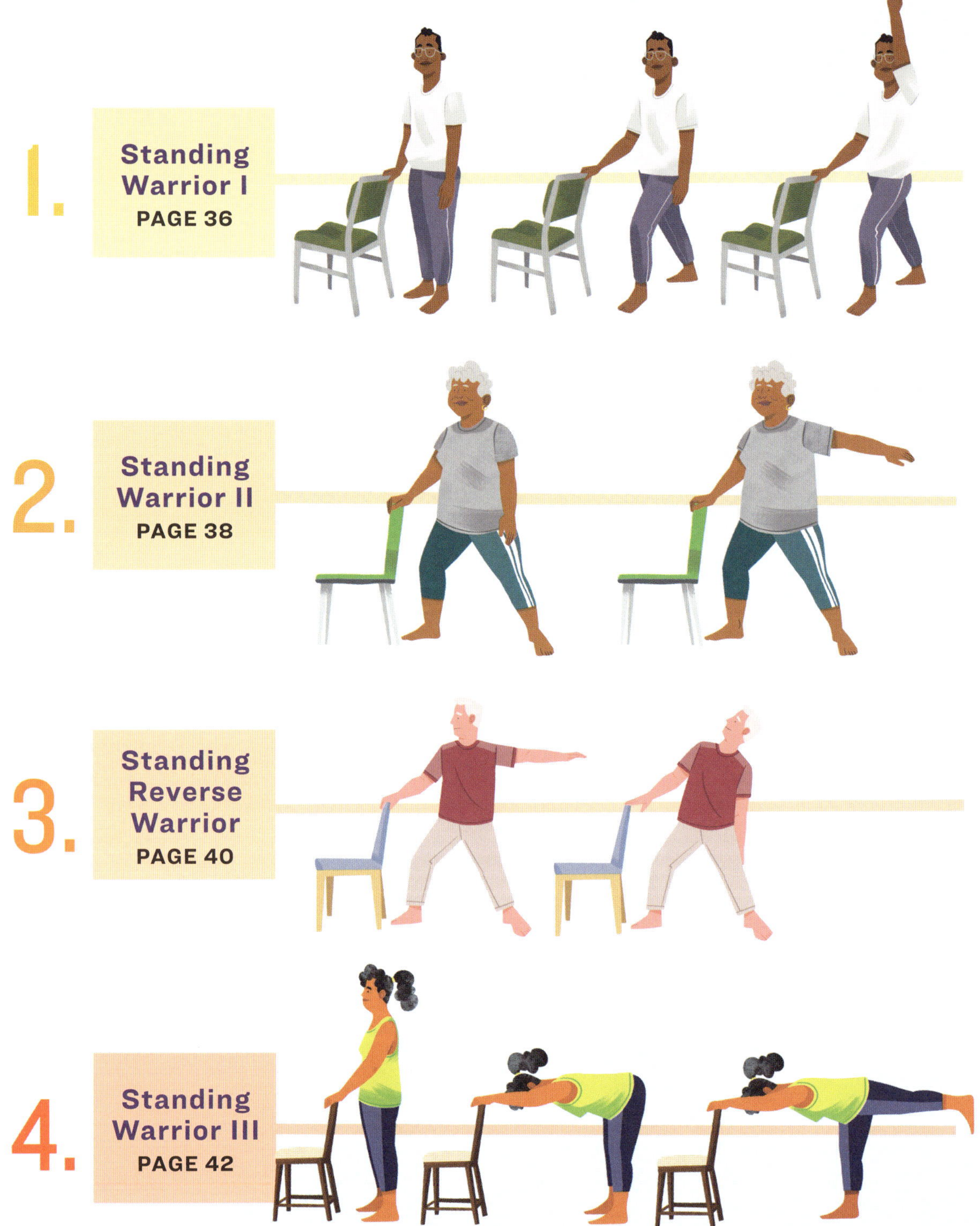
1.
Standing
Warrior I
PAGE 36
2.
Standing
Warrior II
PAGE 38
3.
Standing
Reverse
Warrior
PAGE 40
4.
Standing
Warrior III
PAGE 42

# WARRIOR STRENGTH

**TARGETED BENEFITS:** Balance and Fall Prevention, Mobility and Movement, Muscle Endurance and Strength

Summon your inner gladiator and feel strong, steady, and ready for anything! It's perfect for improving posture and building endurance for daily tasks like carrying groceries, climbing stairs, and gardening. The strength-building poses also support better bone health and reduce the risk of falls. Practice this flow three to four times a week in the morning, or during your day for a muscle-building boost.

## THE SEQUENCE

1. **STANDING WARRIOR I:** Hold for 3 rounds of breath.
2. **STANDING WARRIOR II:** Hold for 3 rounds of breath.
3. **STANDING REVERSE WARRIOR:** Hold for 3 rounds of breath.
4. **STANDING WARRIOR III:** Hold for 3 rounds of breath.
5. Repeat sequence, switching sides with Standing Warrior I, Standing Warrior II, Standing Reverse Warrior, and Standing Warrior III.

**Remember:** Think of your legs as your foundation—strong and supportive. Focus on engaging your muscles as you move and keep your posture tall.

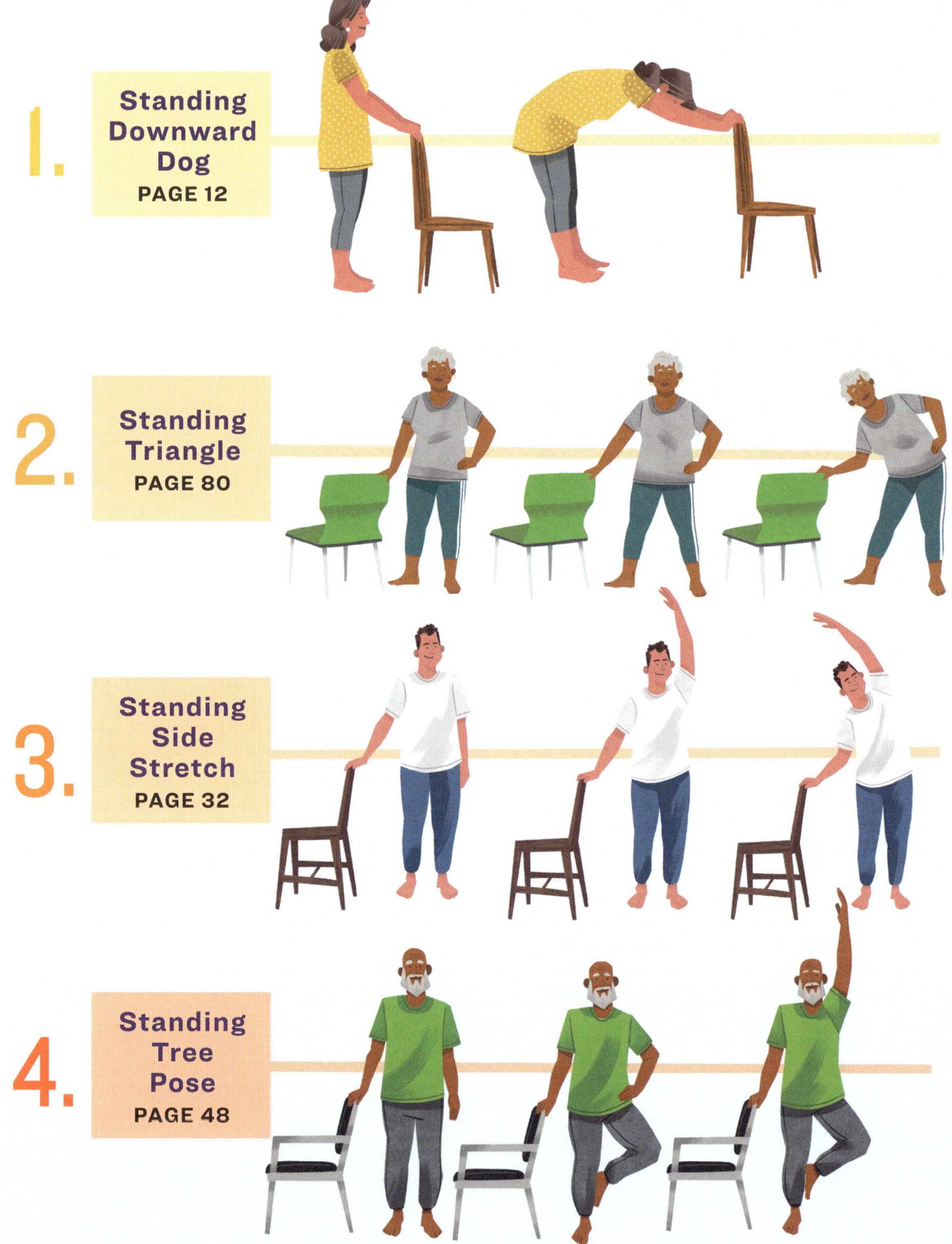
1.
Standing Downward Dog
PAGE 12
2.
Standing Triangle
PAGE 80
3.
Standing Side Stretch
PAGE 32
4.
Standing Tree Pose
PAGE 48

# STANDING BALANCE FLOW

**TARGETED BENEFITS:** Balance and Fall Prevention, Muscle Endurance and Strength

This sequence is perfect for getting your energy flowing before a walk because it will keep you steady on your feet. This sequence strengthens your legs, ankles, and core, giving you the stability needed to handle uneven surfaces or steps with ease. You can also stay connected to your body, bringing mindful intent to your movement. Practice this sequence three times a week.

## THE SEQUENCE

1. **STANDING DOWNWARD DOG:** Do 3 rounds of breath.
2. **STANDING TRIANGLE:** Do 3 rounds of breath.
3. **STANDING SIDE STRETCH:** Do 3 rounds of breath.
4. **STANDING TREE POSE:** Do 3 rounds of breath.
5. Repeat sequence, switching sides with Standing Triangle, Standing Side Stretch, and Standing Tree Pose.

**Remember:** Focus on steady, controlled movements and keep your core engaged to stay balanced. In poses like Standing Downward Dog, let your breath guide you and feel the strength in your legs and arms.

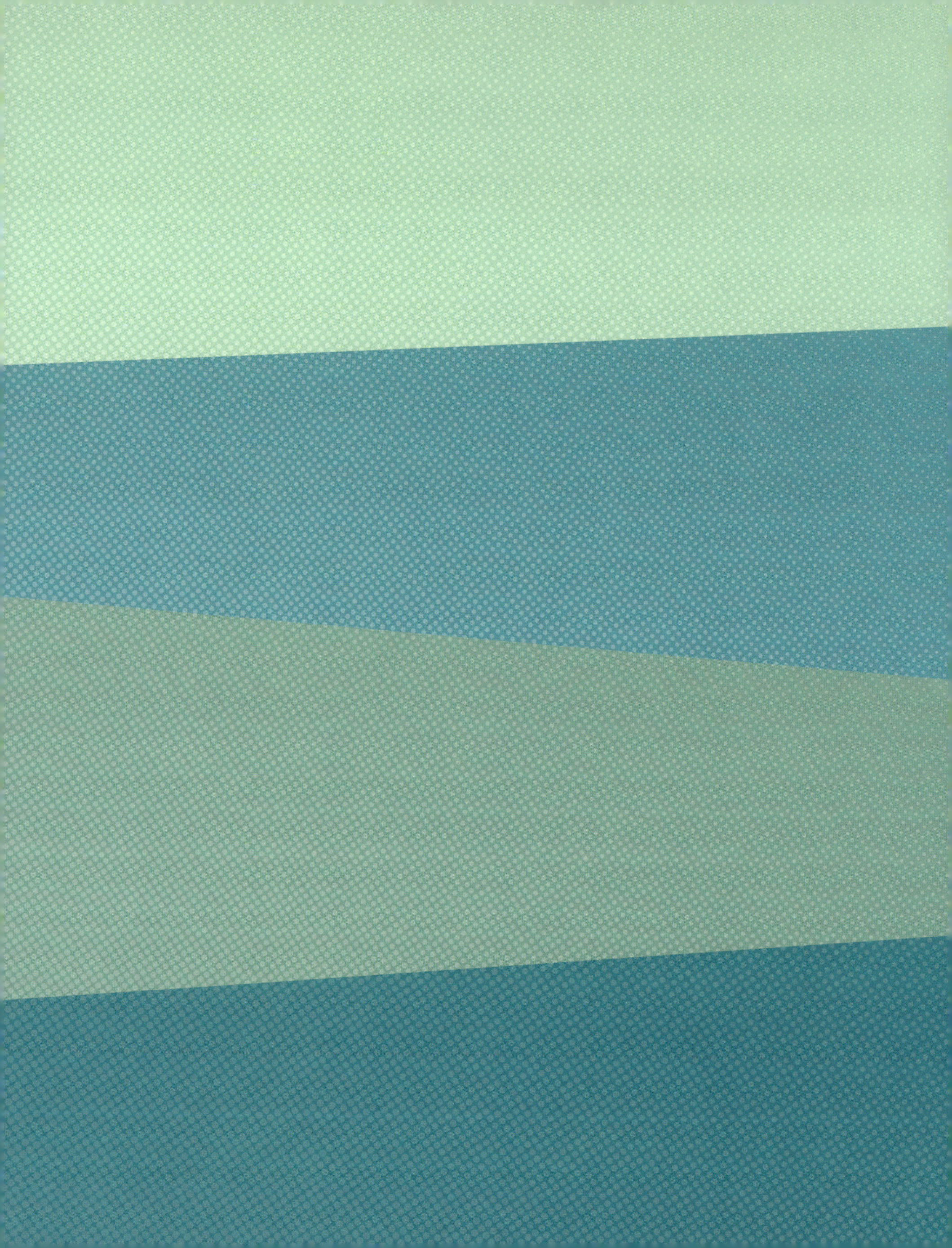

# References

Cramer, Holger, Petra Klose, Benno Brinkhaus, Andreas Michalsen, and Gustav Dobos. "Effects of Yoga on Chronic Neck Pain: A Systematic Review and Meta-Analysis." *Clinical Rehabilitation* 31, no. 11 (March 9, 2017): 1457–65. https://doi.org/10.1177/0269215517698735.

Groessl, Erik J., Lin Liu, Erin L. Richard, and Steven R. Tally. "Cost-Effectiveness of Yoga for Chronic Low Back Pain in Veterans." *Medical Care* 58 (August 13, 2020). https://doi.org/10.1097/mlr.0000000000001356.

Iyengar, B. K. S. *Light on Life: The Yoga Journey to Wholeness, Inner Peace, and Ultimate Freedom*. Emmaus, PA: Rodale, 2005.

Khemani, Sarita. "Stop the Clock: The Shocking Truth about Age-Related Muscle Loss and Steps to Fight Back: Movement & Exercise." Lifestyle Medicine, Stanford University, October 10, 2023. https://lifestylemedicine.stanford.edu/stop-the-clock-the-shocking-truth-about-age-related-muscle-loss-and-steps-to-fight-back.

Krejčí, Milada, Martin Hill, Jiří Kajzar, Miroslav Tichý, and Vaclav Hošek. "Yoga Exercise Intervention Improves Balance Control and Prevents Falls in Seniors Aged 65+." *Slovenian Journal of Public Health* 61, no. 2 (March 21, 2022): 85–92. https://doi.org/10.2478/sjph-2022-0012.

Loewenthal, Julia, Kim E. Innes, Margalit Mitzner, Carol Mita, and Ariela R. Orkaby. “Effect of Yoga on Frailty in Older Adults: A Systematic Review.” *Annals of Internal Medicine* 176, no. 4 (April 2023): 524–35. https://doi.org/10.7326/m22-2553.

“Older Adult Falls Data.” Centers for Disease Control and Prevention. Accessed April 7, 2025. https://www.cdc.gov/falls/data-research/index.html.

“Sarcopenia (Muscle Loss): Symptoms & Causes.” Cleveland Clinic, July 15, 2025. https://my.clevelandclinic.org/health/diseases/23167-sarcopenia.

Skelly, Andrea C., Roger Chou, Joseph R. Dettori, Judith A. Turner, Janna L. Friedly, Sean D. Rundell, Rongwei Fu, et al. “Noninvasive Non-Pharmacological Treatment for Chronic Pain: A Systematic Review Update,” Effective Health Care Program, Agency for Healthcare Research and Quality, April 16, 2020. https://doi.org/10.23970/ahrqepccer227.

Stathokostas, Liza, Matthew W. McDonald, Robert M. Little, and Donald H. Paterson. “Flexibility of Older Adults Aged 55–86 Years and the Influence of Physical Activity.” *Journal of Aging Research* 2013 (2013): 1–8. https://doi.org/10.1155/2013/743843.

Tew, Garry A., Jenny Howsam, Matthew Hardy, and Laura Bissell. “Adapted Yoga to Improve Physical Function and Health-Related Quality of Life in Physically-Inactive Older Adults: A Randomised Controlled Pilot Trial.” *BMC Geriatrics* 17, no. 1 (June 23, 2017). https://doi.org/10.1186/s12877-017-0520-6.

Volpi, Elena, Reza Nazemi, and Satoshi Fujita. “Muscle Tissue Changes with Aging.” Current opinion in clinical nutrition and metabolic care, July 2004. https://pmc.ncbi.nlm.nih.gov/articles/PMC2804956/.

Wang, Man-Ying, Gail A. Greendale, Sean S.-Y. Yu, and George J. Salem. "Physical-performance Outcomes and Biomechanical Correlates from the 32-Week Yoga Empowers Seniors Study." *Evidence-Based Complementary and Alternative Medicine* 2016, no. 1 (January 2016). https://doi.org/10.1155/2016/6921689.

Wang, Yiguo, Shibi Lu, Ruomei Wang, Peng Jiang, Feng Rao, Bo Wang, Yong Zhu, Yihe Hu, and Jianxi Zhu. "Integrative Effect of Yoga Practice in Patients with Knee Arthritis." *Medicine* 97, no. 31 (August 2018). https://doi.org/10.1097/md.0000000000011742.

Wieland, L. Susan, Nicole Skoetz, Karen Pilkington, Ramaprabhu Vempati, Christopher R. D'Adamo, and Brian M. Berman. "Yoga Treatment for Chronic Non-Specific Low Back Pain." *Cochrane Database of Systematic Reviews* 2017, no. 1 (January 12, 2017). https://doi.org/10.1002/14651858.cd010671.pub2.

"Yoga for Arthritis: Benefits of Yoga for the Arthritis Patient." Johns Hopkins Arthritis Center, February 12, 2020. https://www.hopkinsarthritis.org/patient-corner/disease-management/yoga-for-arthritis/.

# Index

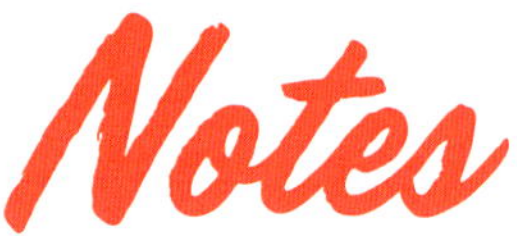
Notes

## ABOUT THE AUTHOR

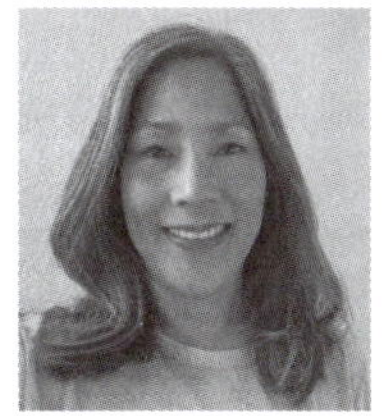

**April Hattori** is the creator of *yes2next* as well as a personal trainer and yoga instructor with certifications from the American Council on Exercise and YogaRenew. On her YouTube channel, she offers free workouts tailored to help people of all ages—especially older adults, beginner exercisers, and those with limited mobility—build strength and improve their health. Connect with her at www.yes2next.com.

## ABOUT THE ILLUSTRATOR

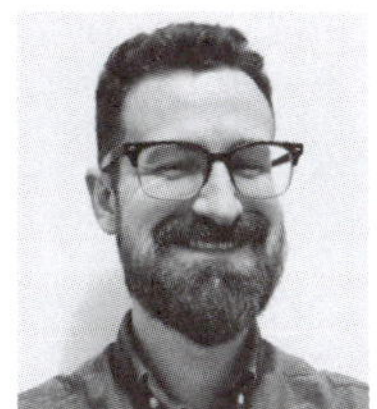

**Drew Bardana** is an illustrator based in Oregon. He creates artwork for brands and publications with rich colors and artful textures. His illustrations often depict lively scenes of people and food, capturing dynamic moments that tell a story. He keeps an active lifestyle to balance the hours spent in the studio. When he's not drawing, you'll find him exploring local hiking trails with his dogs or cooking up healthy recipes in the kitchen. Learn more about Drew at www.drewbardana.com.

# FIND MORE EASY EXERCISES FOR SENIORS WITH THE SERIES!

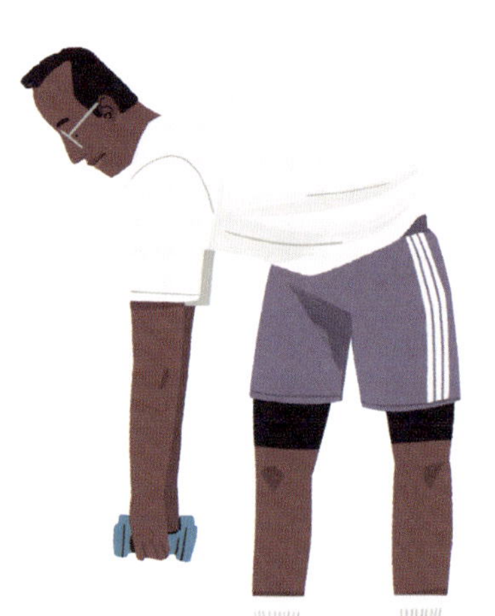

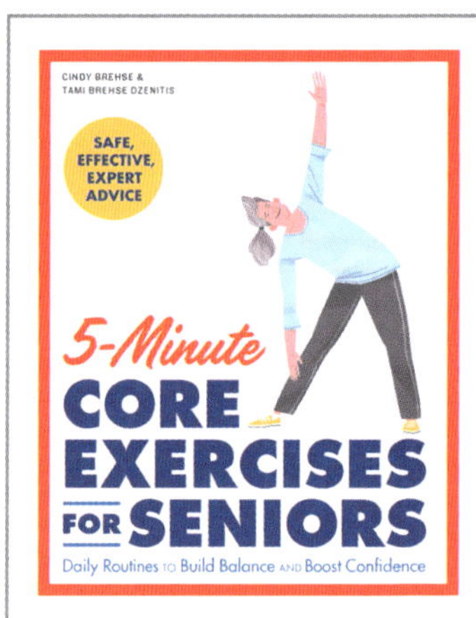


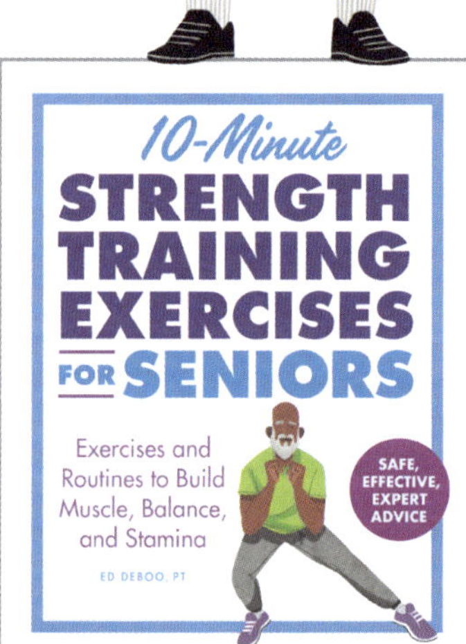


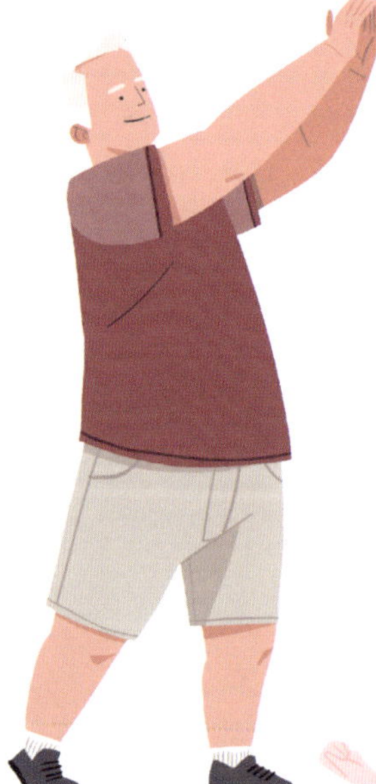

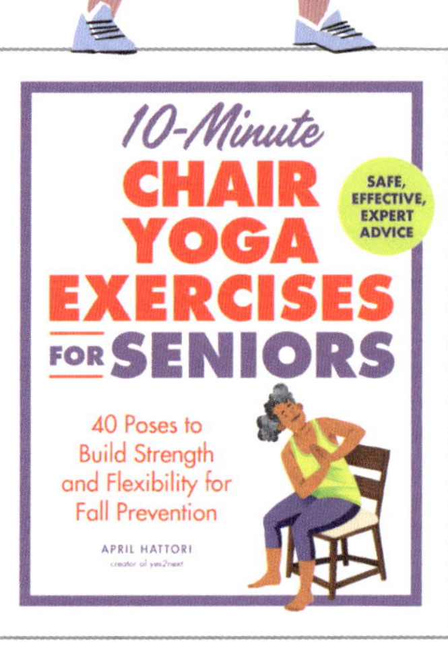


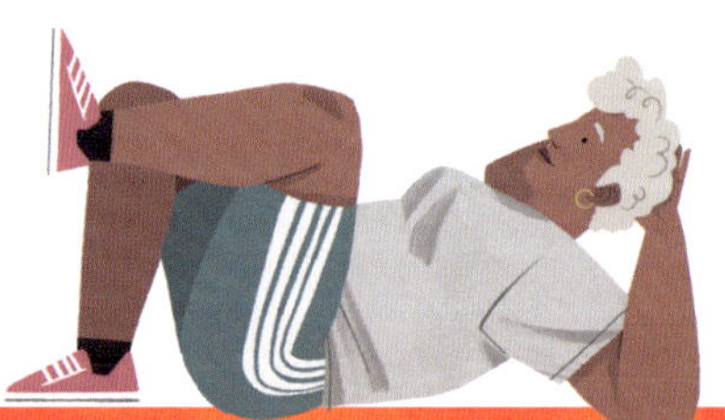